'Howard Levine and his Boston Group were among the first outside of Italy to become interested in the study of post-Bionian Field Theory. Marked by innovative theoretical elaborations and abundant clinical examples, this book is an important testimony to their many fruitful exchanges with Antonino Ferro and the Pavia School. I warmly recommend it to psychotherapists and psychoanalysts at all levels, who are in search of new and versatile working tools to devote to the treatment of psychic suffering.'

– Giuseppe Civitarese, author of *Sublime Subjects: Aesthetic Experience and Intersubjectivity in Psychoanalysis* (Routledge)

'Ferro's integration of Baranger's Field Theory, Bion's theory of transformations and his own concept of co-narratives has had a profound effect on psychoanalysis worldwide. This book shows experienced analysts at work offering readers a clear history, conceptual description, elaboration and clinical application of Ferro's seminal ideas, as it plunges us into zones that are the core of our analytic interactions and psychic life. Levine and the other authors' success in integrating fundamental European, American and South American concepts in their approach makes this book truly unique.'

– Rudi Vermote, author of *Reading Bion* (Routledge), training and supervising analyst, Belgian Psychoanalytic Society

The Post-Bionian Field Theory of Antonino Ferro

This exciting and original collection explores Antonino Ferro's post-Bionian Field Theory, expanding upon the analytic work of Wilfred Bion to focus on the intersubjective development of psychic regulatory processes.

Written by members of the Boston Group for Psychoanalytic Studies who have maintained a close and fruitful collaboration with Ferro and his colleagues, the book centers on understanding, engaging and treating primitive mental states. Ferro's Field Theory operationalizes Bion's concept of an analyst who is not the repository of 'the truth', but is instead one who has the capacity to listen, to dwell in doubt, to utilize reverie, humor and play, and facilitate the transformation of previously unthinkable aspects of the patient's experience into articulatable mental elements such as pictorial images, thoughts and dreams. Ferro's contributions and their analysis are especially relevant to working with primitive character disorders, the difficulties of which lie beyond neurosis and the comfortable reach of the precepts of classical analytic technique.

Each chapter features detailed clinical examples that explicate and apply post-Bionian Field Theory, making this book an interesting and useful read for analysts and analytic therapists of all orientations, who work with patients in all diagnostic categories.

Howard B. Levine is a member of APSA, PINE, the Contemporary Freudian Society, NYU Post-Doc's Contemporary Freudian Track, and is in private practice in Brookline, Massachusetts. He is the author of *Transformations de l'Irreprésentable*, Editor-in-Chief of The Routledge Wilfred R. Bion Studies Book Series and a Director and founding member of the Boston Group for Psychoanalytic Studies.

The Routledge Wilfred R. Bion Studies Book Series

Series Editor Howard B. Levine, MD
Editorial Advisory Board: Nicola Abel-Hirsch, Joseph Aguayo, Avner Bergstein, Lawrence J. Brown, Judith Eekhoff, Claudio Laks Eizerik, Robert D. Hinshelwood, Chris Mawson, James Ogilvie, Elias M. da Rocha Barros, Jani Santamaria, Rudi Vermote

The contributions of Wilfred Bion are among the most cited in the analytic literature. Their appeal lies not only in their content and explanatory value, but in their generative potential. Although Bion's training and many of his clinical instincts were deeply rooted in the classical tradition of Melanie Klein, his ideas have a potentially universal appeal. Rather than emphasizing a particular psychic content (e.g., Oedipal conflicts in need of resolution; splits that needed to be healed; preconceived transferences that must be allowed to form and flourish, etc.), he tried to help open and prepare the mind of the analyst (without memory, desire or theoretical preconception) for the encounter with the patient.

Bion's formulations of group mentality and the psychotic and non-psychotic portions of the mind, his theory of thinking and emphasis on facing and articulating the truth of one's existence so that one might truly learn first hand from one's own experience, his description of psychic development (alpha function and container/contained) and his exploration of **O** are "non-denominational" concepts that defy relegation to a particular school or orientation of psychoanalysis. Consequently, his ideas have taken root in many places ... and those ideas continue to inform many different branches of psychoanalytic inquiry and interest.[1]

It is with this heritage and its promise for the future developments of psychoanalysis in mind that we present *The Routledge Wilfred R. Bion Studies Book Series*. This series gathers together under newly emerging and continually evolving contributions to psychoanalytic thinking that rest upon Bion's foundational texts and explore and extend the implications of his thought.

For a full list of titles in the series, please visit the Routledge website at: https://www.routledge.com/The-Routledge-Wilfred-Bion-Studies-Book-Series/book-series/RWBSBS

---

[1] Levine, H.B. and Civitarese, G. (2016). Editors' Preface, *The W. R. Bion Tradition*, Levine and Civitarese, eds, London: Karnac 2016, p. xxi.

The Post-Bionian Field Theory of Antonino Ferro

Theoretical Analysis and Clinical Application

Edited by
Howard B. Levine

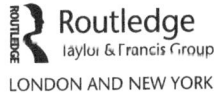
Routledge
Taylor & Francis Group

LONDON AND NEW YORK

First published 2022
by Routledge
2 Park Square, Milton Park, Abingdon, Oxon OX14 4RN

and by Routledge
605 Third Avenue, New York, NY 10158

Routledge is an imprint of the Taylor & Francis Group, an informa business

© 2022 selection and editorial matter, Howard B. Levine; individual chapters, the contributors

British Library Cataloguing-in-Publication Data
A catalogue record for this book is available from the British Library

Library of Congress Cataloging-in-Publication Data
Names: Levine, Howard B., editor.
Title: The post-Bionian field theory of Antonino Ferro : theoretical analysis and clinical application / [edited by] Howard B. Levine.
Description: Abingdon, Oxon ; New York, NY : Routledge, 2022. |
Series: The Routledge Wilfred R. Bion studies book series | Includes bibliographical references. |
Summary: "This exciting and original collection explores Antonino Ferro's Post-Bionian Field Theory, expanding upon the analytic work of Wilfred Bion to focus on the inter-subjective development of psychic regulatory processes. Each chapter features detailed clinical examples that explicate and apply Post-Bionian Field Theory, making this book an interesting and useful read for analysts and analytic therapists of all orientations, who work with patients in all diagnostic categories"-- Provided by publisher.
Identifiers: LCCN 2021030886 (print) | LCCN 2021030887 (ebook) |
ISBN 9780367766740 (hardback) | ISBN 9780367766733 (paperback) |
ISBN 9781003168034 (ebook)
Subjects: LCSH: Ferro, Antonino, 1947- | Bion, Wilfred R. (Wilfred Ruprecht), 1897-1979. | Psychiatry. | Psychoanalysis.
Classification: LCC RC506 .P6244 2022 (print) | LCC RC506 (ebook) |
DDC 616.89/17--dc23
LC record available at https://lccn.loc.gov/2021030886
LC ebook record available at https://lccn.loc.gov/2021030887

ISBN: 978-0-367-76674-0 (hbk)
ISBN: 978-0-367-76673-3 (pbk)
ISBN: 978-1-003-16803-4 (ebk)

DOI: 10.4324/9781003168034

Typeset in Times New Roman
by Taylor & Francis Books

'Psychoanalysis is not a symbolic system charged with "deciphering meaning", but a "system for generating new thoughts".'

(Ferro, *Psychoanalysis as Therapy and Storytelling*, 2006, p. 92)

Contents

Contributors

Rodrigo Barahona is a psychoanalyst in private practice in Brookline, Massachusetts, a Director of the Boston Group for Psychoanalytic Studies (BGPS), a faculty member of the Boston Psychoanalytic Society and Institute where he has taught on the subjects of Bion and psychopathology, serves on numerous editorial boards and is the Book Review Editor of the *Psychoanalytic Quarterly.*

Lawrence J. Brown is a graduate of the Boston Psychoanalytic Institute (BPSI) in both Child and Adult Psychoanalysis, a Supervising Child Analyst and recent Co-Chair of the Child Analysis program at BPSI. He is on the Editorial Board of the *Psychoanalytic Quarterly* and is President of BGPS. His book, *Intersubjective Processes and the Unconscious: An Integration of Freudian, Kleinian and Bionian Perspectives,* was published in 2011 by Routledge. He also co-edited two other recent books: *Growth and Turbulence in the Container/Contained: Bion's Continuing Legacy* (with Howard Levine; Routledge, 2013); and *On Freud's 'Formulations on the Two Principles of Mental Functioning'* (with Gabriela Legorreta; Karnac Books, 2016). His latest book, *Transformational Processes in Clinical Psychoanalysis: Dreaming, Emotions and the Present Moment,* was published in 2018 by IPA Publications and Routledge. He is currently editing a book of essays, *Commentaries on Freud's Moses and Monotheism,* which will be published by Routledge.

Howard B. Levine is a founding Director of BGPS, a member of PINE, the Contemporary Freudian Society, on the faculty of NYU Post-Doc's Contemporary Freudian Track, on the Editorial Board of the *International Journal of Psychoanalysis* and *Psychoanalytic Inquiry,* Editor-in-Chief of The Routledge Wilfred R. Bion Studies Book Series and in private practice in Brookline, Massachusetts. He is the author of *Transformations de l'Irreprésentable* (2019) and the forthcoming *Affect, Representation and Language: Between the Silence and the Cry* (Routledge). His co-edited books include *Unrepresented States and the Construction of Meaning* (Karnac, 2013); *On Freud's Screen Memories* (Karnac, 2014); *The Wilfred Bion Tradition* (Karnac, 2016); *Bion in Brazil*

(Karnac, 2017); and *Andre Green Revisited: Representation and the Work of the Negative* (Karnac, 2018).

Allen Palmer is a Board member of BGPS, a supervising and training analyst and a child supervising analyst at the Boston Psychoanalytic Society and Institute (BPSI), former Chairperson of the Supervising and Training Analyst Committee and of the Child Psychoanalysis Program and an active faculty member in the Joint Child and Adult Psychoanalytic Training Program at BPSI. He practices adult, child and adolescent psychotherapy and psychoanalysis and supervision in Newton Highlands, Massachusetts.

David G. Power is a founding Director of BGPS, Past President, Supervisory and Teaching Analyst at the Massachusetts Institute for Psychoanalysis, on the faculty of the Boston Psychoanalytic Society and Institute and is an Instructor in Psychology in the Department of Psychiatry (PT), Harvard Medical School at Cambridge Health Alliance. He is co-editor with Howard Levine of *Engaging Primitive Anxieties of the Emerging Self* (Karnac, 2017) and maintains a private practice in psychoanalysis, psychotherapy and supervision in Cambridge, Massachusetts.

Dolan Power is a founding Director of BGPS, Past President, Supervisory and Teaching Analyst at the Massachusetts Institute for Psychoanalysis and on the Faculty of the Boston Psychoanalytic Society and Institute. She was awarded the Francis Tustin Memorial Prize in 2011 for her paper 'The use of the analyst as an autistic shape' published in 2016 in the *International Journal of Psychoanalysis*. She maintains a private practice in psychoanalysis, consultation and supervision in Cambridge, Massachusetts.

Preface

The Boston Group for Psychoanalytic Studies (BGPS) is a non-profit psycho-analytic educational organization founded in 2007 by a group of friends and colleagues, who shared a common interest in creating psychoanalytic educational opportunities for themselves and for colleagues that could extend beyond the standard subjects or theories then being taught in the Boston area. BGPS grew out of the organizing committee for the international Bion in Boston Conference held in 2009 in Boston, MA. With an original target audience of recent graduates, mid-career analysts and advanced candidates, BGPS has gone on to sponsor seminars, lectures and small-group clinical discussions for analysts and analytic therapists of all levels, and on many subjects including British Object Relations Theory (Kleinian, Winnicottian and Independent), Contemporary French Psychoanalysis (Andre Green, Patrick Miller, Marilia Aisenstein and the Paris Psychosomatic School), Bionian Field Theory and currents in contemporary Latin American psychoanalysis. In addition, BGPS sponsored the 7th International Conference on the Work of Frances Tustin in 2014 and participated in helping to organize the first Bion in Marrakech conference in 2012.

Our relationship with Nino Ferro, Giuseppe Civitarese and their colleagues at the Pavia branch of the Italian Society (SPI) has been longstanding, warm and mutually rewarding. We have hosted and worked with Nino, Giuseppe and Roberto Basile in Boston, some of us have visited Pavia and worked with Nino and colleagues there, and many have met and worked together at international conferences and congresses. Field Theory has been an important topic of discussion among the Board members of BGPS and has taken root clinically and theoretically in our minds and work. It has deeply influenced many of our colleagues and conference participants as well. It is therefore fitting that several of us have come together to consider where we stand in relation to its influences and to share those considerations with you, our readers. We hope that you will find this topic and our efforts as worthwhile and thought provoking as we have.

Howard B. Levine, MD
BGPS

Foreword

Antonino Ferro

This book arises out of the encounter between what we can call an expansion of late Bion and the final version of the Field Theory. The precipitation and conjoining of these ideas owes much to the 2009 International Bion Conference in Boston.

It seems to me that Howard Levine and his co-authors have succeeded in navigating some highly complex concepts and making them their own, bringing them to the reader metabolized and energized. In particular, they take on the challenge of describing and narrating the most complex angles of Bionian Field Theory in an extremely clear way. I could say that the authors act constantly as an alpha function capable of 'alphabetizing' certain still obscure passages of theory and technique, making them dreamable and thus comprehensible. The clinical examples that are provided are always brilliant and simple, capable of making a difficult theory accessible. I believe I myself will be one of the beneficiaries of this work, which continually expands the field that it explores. A book which seemed to offer itself as a summary of certain theories becomes a catalyst and generator of thoughts. The reader is transported into Bion's way of thinking, conjoined with Field Theories: Bionian Field Theory comes to life in this union.

What is revolutionary in Bion's thought lies in its having postulated the existence of a continual day-dreaming which constantly alphabetizes all the sensoriality (and obscurity) that pervades us, building a chain which leads from alpha elements to pictograms, to waking dream thought, and to the perennial construction of an unconscious by the Field's alpha function. This is the result of a kind of Big Bang which comes into being every time analyst and patient meet, bringing continually expanding multi-verses to life. With Grotstein, before his death, we had theorized the existence of a super-alpha-function which, by using what the diurnal alpha function had stored away, would bring the nocturnal dream to life. Howard Levine has been able to reconstruct and illuminate these long and complex paths, showing its various levels of organization and underlining not only its origin in Bion and the field, but also what it has drawn from Kleinian Theory and French psycho-analysis, giving a fully rounded, finished product which on the one hand allows access to a metabolized product and on the other offers new starting points for thought. In its variously articulated marriage with Field Theory, the oneiric shows the development of a theory in a constant state of becoming. The field becomes ill with the patient's illness; and it is in the field that the tools for thinking, dreaming and feeling (alpha function, container/contained, negative capability, selected fact) are developed. Narrative, storytelling, and the development of a container are seen as key points of a kind of oneiric orchestra in development. I'd like to be able to comment 1:1, but that would mean rewriting the entire book!

So, I must make do with underlining some particularly vivid points. Special appreciation should be given to the direct use of clinical material: on the one hand we navigate the maps of the theory, and on the other we navigate the turbulent sea of clinical situations that enable us to discover all the strategies for continually tuning the analytic instruments. The signs coming from the field, transformations in dream, oneiric flashes, and the world of reveries are further material constantly coming to the boil and indicating speculative new paths. It's wonderful to see how the field expands thanks also to the personal contributions of Levine and his co-authors. The web's narrative network oscillates and expands, and at the same time gives some starting points which allow narratively significant developments, such as the characters who hide and are transformed in the field: human characters, but also characters that are atmospheres or emotions, and (why not?) objects. The author's writing often reminds me of Italo Calvino in its simplicity and depth, especially his *American Lectures* and *The Castle of Crossed Destinies* where new stories are formed by the interplay of tarot cards.

I would also like to stress the pleasure to be had from reading this book and especially the irony and occasional comedy brought out by many of the stories, making the text lively and exciting.

The book plumbs the primitive states of alpha work and the very early activities that are a prelude to the formation of alpha elements and pictograms. Their specific characteristics are explored in Bionian Field Theory along with the similarities and differences with the outlooks of Piera Aulagnier and Elias Rocha Barros. And so, many early states are used to explore reverie and the *betalomas* (as Barale and I [1992] have called the aggregations of beta elements).

The book draws on the thinking of Bion and Winnicott to address the importance of the corporeal register and the circulation and elaboration of projective identifications in the field. We should remember the central importance of Bion's contribution to understanding the origin of thinking. The characters, their articulation in a narrative, their transformations in dream, play and hallucinosis, create a new theoretical space. I think that, by its nature, theory should be a bit obscure, or rather a bit hazy. Here, Ogden's ideas fit with, and often clarify, such narrative theoretical cruxes because of his extraordinary capacity for making bold new concepts accessible – *talking as dreaming* (Ogden, 2007), for example – and the way he has clarified the understanding of analysis as either *epistemological* or *ontological* (2019).

A key point highlighted at various points in the text is the transition from a theory and technique based on interpretation to a theory and technique whose pillars are transformations. Negative capability is that medium which enables and fosters transformations in play and dream, and leads towards the 'O' of the field's evolution. Ideas that have found a broad development in psychoanalysis had previously been elaborated in philosophy, especially in those German authors leading to K. Lewin.

It is also important to see how the internal groupality of patient and analyst may lead to a multi-groupality which comes to life in the field itself, giving life in turn to the oscillation between *Characters in search of authors* and *Authors in search of characters* (Pirandello, 1995 [1925]). The oneiric factor is also fundamental in child analysis, where I started with *The Bipersonal Field* (1992) and, before that, Kancyper had stressed how parents and siblings also belong to the field. Here too there is a reversal of perspective in terms of thinking about the narrated parents, as well as the really existing ones, as characters who enable the narration/explication of field-functions which demand to be narrated. In this way, parents, teachers, partners become characters of the field who embody emotions and ways of functioning that are waiting for actors who might bring them onto the stage thanks to the work of *casting agents* (Larry Brown, this volume).

With its characteristics of depth and expansion, the field naturally leads to the co-presence within it of reverie, negative reverie, alpha function, and inverted alpha function: in other words, if we wanted to refer to a Grid of the field, we would have to reckon with its Negative Grid as well; not only with the expansion of the negative (Green, 1999) but also with the study of still unexplored modes of functioning of the field and the two minds.

This book allows new pathways to open up towards ways of functioning which have not yet become part of our theoretical–clinical heritage. What I would call the unsaturatedness of the text provides a kind of master key for the not-yet-thought which is the most eagerly sought goal of our researches. I thank Howard Levine and his co-authors for having dared to open up new routes for us to navigate and invite our readers to join us in this adventure.

References

Barale, F. and Ferro, A. (1992). Negative therapeutic reactions and microfractures in analytic communication. In *Shared Experience: The Psychoanalytic Dialogue*. Ed. by L. Nissim and A. Robutti. London: Karnac Books. pp. 143–165.

Ferro, A. (1992). *The Bipersonal Field: Experiences in Child Analysis*. London and New York: Routledge.

Green, A. (1999). *The Work of the Negative*. London: Free Association Books.

Ogden, T.H. (2007). On talking as dreaming. *International Journal of Psychoanalysis*, 88 (3): 575–589.

Ogden, T.H. (2019). Ontological psychoanalysis or 'What do you want to be when you grow up?' *The Psychoanalytic Quarterly*, 88 (4): 661–684.

Pirandello, L. (1995 [1925]). *Six Characters in Search of an Author*. London: Penguin Books.

Chapter 1

The transformational vision of Antonino Ferro[1]

Howard B. Levine

I like to think of the analyst ... as a great storyteller, who knows how to bring to life narremes and stories of the patient and of the field, and is free to detach himself from his psychoanalytic knowledge in order to sail beyond the Pillars of Hercules, beyond the psychoanalytically known, towards new worlds of unthought thinkability and the thoughts in search of a thinker that await us in the Americas of the mind.

(Ferro, 2006, p. 6)

Introduction

In 1979, at the conclusion of his Italian Seminars, Bion (2005) left his audience with an evocative image of uncertainty and poetic beauty, when he compared his contribution to the seminars to a leaf falling from a tree: 'One never knows which side up it will land' (p. 104). He then challenged his listeners by asking, 'What is this group likely to give birth to? What thought or idea or action? And what relationship is likely to occur between it and some other group? Love or hate? Fight or flight? Dependence or freedom?' (p. 104).

At the 2009 IPA Congress in Chicago, Parisi (2009) looked back over the preceding 30 years and suggested that Bion's influence on Italian psychoanalysis has been both widespread and profound. In her view, in contrast to the then more established European analytic societies, Bion's ideas, especially the more innovative thought of his later years, gained widespread acceptance 'perhaps because [they] arrived at the right time to give space to call for authenticity in a group who had just recently formed, and who clearly needed to start feeling themselves freer from rigid elements of theory' (Parisi, 2009).

Nowhere are the fruits of this influence and encouragement of freedom of thought more evident than in the work of Antonino Ferro. Although not present at Bion's seminars in Rome, Ferro has proven to be among the most fertile, productive and creative of his descendants, the embodiment of Bion's

DOI: 10.4324/9781003168034-1

concept of

> an analyst who was not the repository of the truth, but rather had the capacity to listen, to dwell on doubts, to utilize his own capacity for reverie to get in touch with his own unconscious [and that of the patient] and therefore transform the unthinkable aspects of the patient's experience.
>
> (Parisi, 2009)

into articulatable mental elements: i.e. pictorial images, thoughts and dreams.

Like Bion, Ferro sees the work of analysis as facilitating patients' capacities for *being* rather than just *knowing about*, a being that implies creativity in the understanding and construction of one's identity and life trajectory. However, Ferro's view of the analyst as catalyst and co-constructor of the patients' narrative develops what is only implicit in Bion's writings, in its formulation of the analyst's role in helping patients 'expand and develop their capacities to tolerate and represent thoughts and feelings and elaborate them into narrative sequences' (Levine, 2006, p. 673). As they do so, patients enlarge their unconscious and organize and structure their psyches, as they increase their tolerance for and achieve closer contact with previously non-negotiable areas of their minds.

This is a catalytic, *transformational* vision of psychoanalysis, which Ferro could arrive at only after transcending what he experienced as a rigid and doctrinaire application of classical Kleinian training. In his view (Ferro, 2002a, especially pp. 13–32), the latter placed so much emphasis on the analyst's attempting to know, decode and interpret the contents of the patient's unconscious, that it risked creating a persecutory atmosphere within the analytic relationship. What helped Ferro move beyond its strictures was a deep appreciation of Bion's emphasis on the receptivity of the analyst's mind as a key component of an interactive, intersubjective analytic process and Bion's subordination of the classical Freudian objectives of recovering psychic *contents* (e.g. repressed childhood memories and unacceptable (to the superego) wishes and desires) and reworking and resolving psychic conflict to the broader aim of helping catalyze the expansion and creation of the patient's mind.[2] Thus, Ferro's fondness for Bion's (1970) emphasis on the here-and-now of the analytic moment and assertion that psychoanalysis is a probe that expands the very domain it seeks to explore.[3]

In addition to Bion, Ferro also drew upon the work of Winnicott (especially the Squiggle Game, developmental facilitation and the importance of non-interpretive therapeutic factors), Willi and Madeleine Baranger (2009) (intersubjectivity and the analytic Field), his training and experience as a child analyst, and Italian literary sources such as Luigi Pirandello (author of the play *Six Characters in Search of an Author*, who famously declared that 'the truth is a blur in motion') and Umberto Eco (narratology). The result is a vision of psychoanalysis that is playful, intuitive, spontaneous and, above all, transformational. Since many North American readers are still not easily conversant with Bion's theory or comfortable with the language in which it is written, a 'dialect' that Ferro uses easily and fluently in his own writings, I will begin with a synopsis of Bion's work presented with Ferro's use of Bion in mind.

Bion

Bion favored the fostering of individual creativity over the indoctrination of disciples[4] and insisted that he did not wish to have people try to analyze as he did. Rather, he tried to tell them something of how he believed that *he* did analysis, in the hopes that they might learn something more about how they believed that *they* did analysis. His interest was deeply rooted in the relationship that exists between the mind of the patient and the mind of the analyst and he is known, among other things, for his 'theory of thinking' (Bion, 1962a). He advanced the view that the only material for which the analyst has direct evidence is his or her subjective emotional experience of the analytic sessions (Bion, 1970). All the rest, the patient's past history, descriptions of extra-analytic interactions, etc., he called 'hearsay evidence', which he felt was of limited value. Thus, for Bion, the here-and-now of the session, especially the state and functioning of the mind of the analyst and its degree of receptivity to the projections and needs of the patient, forms the fundamental reality of the psychoanalytic situation and serves as a central locus of analytic investigation.[5]

With these assumptions as his starting points, Bion tried in his writings and lectures to prepare the minds of analysts for their encounters with their patients. In particular, he sought to direct analysts' attention to the immediate, emerging experience of the here-and-now, in the hopes that they might thereby discern the impact on the patient and the analytic relationship of an unknowable unconscious reality. Thus, Bion encouraged analysts to be receptive to their patient's projections, with the latter viewed not only as defenses, evacuations and phantasied attempts at aggressive assault and omnipotent control as Freud and Klein had seen them, but also as primitive attempts at communication and covert appeals for containment and transformation of what was overwhelming and unmanageable for the patient.

For Bion, primitive mental states (often referred to as or associated with 'the psychotic part of the mind') did not lend themselves to expression through language and verbalization. Rather, they 'announced their presence' (communicated) by inducing emotions in the analyst, which were covert attempts for intersubjective assistance in containment and metabolization of otherwise uncontrollable and potentially traumatic affects and forces.

In order to absorb, recognize and therefore have a chance of being able to metabolize these projections, Bion felt that the analyst must encounter the patient at every moment without preconceptions ('without memory or desire'), tolerate the frustration and ambiguity of not knowing while one waits for meaning to emerge ('negative capability') and allow for and cultivate a capacity for spontaneous and intuitive response. Eschewing the expectation of discovering and decoding pre-determined mental contents (e.g. derivatives of the Oedipus complex, childhood traumata or the defensive activity of the ego), he focused instead upon analysis as a process that was highly original, wide ranging, pair-specific, dialogic, creative and deeply intersubjective.

Central to Bion's (1962b, 1970) thinking was the assumption that the mental activity that produces nighttime dreams also takes place while we are awake.[6] In the latter instance, what the dream work produces is unconscious 'waking dream thoughts' made from the building blocks of representational mental life that Bion called 'alpha elements'. This activity is seen as vital, omnipresent and essential for psychic homeostasis and therefore adaptation, because in Bion's view, existence, in its raw, unprocessed, unrepresented and unrepresentable form, is overwhelming and potentially traumatic. Note that as Ferro (2002b) has described, Bion

> turns Freud's position on dreams upside down: whereas Freud used the term 'dreamwork' to mean that otherwise incomprehensible unconscious material was transformed into dreams and that the dreamwork had to be undone in order to make the incomprehensible dream comprehensible again (Freud, 1933), Bion thinks that conscious material has to be subjected to dreamwork to render it suitable for storing away and for thought.
>
> (p. 598)

The term that Bion gave to raw, unprocessed data is 'beta elements'. These are inchoate, 'proto-psychic' somatic and sensorial sensations that are registered somatically, but not psychically represented in any way that we ordinarily think of as 'psychological'.[7] The fact that beta elements are proto- or extra-psychic means that they cannot be recognized, articulated, used to form thoughts or to think with or think about, unless and until they are transformed and made into something psychological. The process through which this transformation occurs is called 'alpha function'. It begins with the formation of visual 'pictograms'[8] (alpha elements) from vague visceral and perceptual sensations and is the constant activity through which the psyche transforms ('metabolizes') the raw data (beta elements) of internal and external sensation and perception into something that is discernible and usable by the mind as the building blocks of symbolically and emotionally invested thought.

Beta elements, like the drives in Freud's theory, are analogous to subatomic particles in a cloud chamber. The impacts and disturbances caused by their presence can be noted, but they cannot be directly observed. Thus, while beta elements do register and create impacts, what we colloquially call 'experience' – something that is noticeable and capable of being reflected upon and understood in a cause-and-effect sequence or chain of events – may only come into being after beta elements have been transformed into alpha elements. Once alpha elements are created, either by the action of one's own alpha function or the alter ego-like functioning of the alpha function of another (e.g. mother, analyst), they can then be linked into symbolic chains and strung together in narrative sequences in the psyche by additional mental processes that Bion calls 'the apparatus for thinking thoughts' and 'the apparatus for dreaming dreams' and Ferro calls 'narrative function'.

Whether sensations arise from internal or external sources, i.e. originate as drives or perceptions, Bion assumed that they were inherently chaotic and potentially traumatic and so required processing and transformation ('metabolization'), if one was to emotionally survive the turbulence that they produced. His description of the individual constantly bombarded by beta elements and faced with the problem of how to withstand the very act of perception is not dissimilar to how Freud viewed the problem of the psyche *vis-à-vis* the drives.

In his metapsychology papers, Freud (1911, 1915a, 1915b) hypothesized that the Unconscious – later the Id (Freud, 1923) – consisted in large part of unbound pressures and energies ('thing presentations') that had to be 'tamed' by language – (given content and limited in meaning by being united with 'word presentations') – in order to prevent traumatic disruption of mental processes and reach articulation and potential consciousness. Thus, Freud said the drives make a demand upon the psyche for work – i.e. the psyche must expend energy and do work on the drive derivatives in order to give them form and content and help them achieve representation in the mind. Freud's emphasis on the importance of 'taming' the drives raised the problems of representation and non-representation to the center of metapsychological and clinical importance.

An analogous argument can be made for Bion in terms of each individual's need to develop sufficient capacity for alpha function, so as to protect themselves from and tame the continual assault of beta elements. Indeed, for Bion the regulatory, homeostatic need to create psychic (alpha) elements that are symbolically invested and capable of being represented in the mind is almost an evolutionary biological *raison d'etre* for the mental apparatus. Thus, while Freud's famous summation of the clinical goal of psychoanalysis was: 'Where id was there ego shall be', for Bion, we might say: 'Where beta was, there alpha shall be' or even more broadly: 'Where chaos was, there order and psychic structure shall be'.

Once sufficient psychic representation has taken place, we can then begin to talk about and observe symbolically and emotionally invested thoughts linked together into chains of associations and the ordinary rules of classical analytic technique may apply. Even then, however, each of us is continually subjected to an onslaught of new beta elements. This means that each of us possesses an inexhaustible potential for the creation of new thoughts that can be activated by the analytic relationship and interlinked into a broad, almost infinite variety of narrative descriptions. It also means that each of us is faced with the potential distress caused by an excess of 'undigested' beta elements and may be in need of the relief that can only come from the intervention of another (e.g. the analyst or mother). The kind of intervention that Bion had in mind was dependent upon the analyst's (mother's) using his or her alpha function in the service of the patient's (infant's) regulatory needs. This requires – and begins with – an optimal state of receptivity to the patient's projections on the analyst's part, so that they may be absorbed by the analyst, worked upon and transformed into alpha elements, strung together into meaningful thoughts that can then be thought and reflected upon by the analyst and used as the basis for an appropriate analytic response and/or intervention.

In order to achieve this optimal state of absorption and receptivity, the analyst is asked to be in a state of *reverie*, without memory, desire or intention. As much as possible, this is a state of pure receptivity and negative capability that

> implies the existence of an on-going emotional exchange within the analytic couple, in which proto-emotions, proto-sensations – beta elements – can be evacuated by the patient and then collected by the analyst's mind, which is capable of transforming and elaborating them.
>
> (Ferro, 2005b, p. 424)

In this process, the analyst represents these elements with and in a sense *for* the patient in his or her own mind and then 're-presents'[9] them to the patient, who can then use them to form the elements of thought. In this process of reverie-absorption-transformation-representation-re-presentation, which Bion called '*container/contained*', the patient (or developing infant and child) also introjects and/or develops the capacity [=alpha function] for accomplishing this kind of transformation on his or her own.

What this means practically is that we try to enter the session without preconceptions about what should or will happen or what we need to talk about. We don't try to recall the patient's history, worry about what happened in the last session, how it may or may not fit into the theory we are learning or what our last formulation or our supervisor has directed our attention to in the previous hours. We wait to see what occurs, including what spontaneously occurs to us, and try to see it in the here-and-now. At times, what spontaneously occurs to the analyst may be a memory (e.g. of what happened last time) or a desire (e.g. that such-and-such should happen). These are spontaneous occurrences are not the 'memory and desire' that Bion warns us against. They are reflections of the 'now' of the moment (what Bion (1970) calls 'O') and arise unbidden in the session, rather than being carried into the session as pre-conceptions artificially brought in from the outside. As spontaneous occurrences, they should be valued for their communicative value as important reflections of the analytic moment.

Bion had a strong belief in the *communicative function of projective identification* (Spillius, 1992) and so encouraged analysts to take whatever occurred to them in the session or when thinking or dreaming about the patient – what he called 'making room for wild thoughts' – as a potential channel of information about the analytic process and relationship and to consider how such thoughts might fit into and offer perspectives upon the current analytic situation. Ogden (1994), for example, has made good use of this injunction in his development of the clinical implications of 'the analytic third' and Botella and Botella (2005) have described how the intuitive, spontaneous comment or action that catalyzes an act of *figurability* in the patient may often begin in the mind of the analyst as an eruptive impulse (e.g. 'wild thought'). In relation to classical formulations, these wild thoughts may reflect, at the same time, both the traditional countertransference, when viewed from the perspective of the analyst's psychic conflicts and functioning, and a source of feedback about the analytic situation, when viewed from the perspective of the Field (see below). As Bion might say, how they appear is a function of the 'vertex' (perspective) from which they are being observed.

By encouraging us to make room for wild thoughts, Bion did not mean to endorse indiscriminate self-revelation or wild analysis. His recommendation followed from his conviction that the unconscious minds of patient and analyst combined to form a dyadic, intersubjective unit – which he called a 'group of two' or 'thinking couple'. One can see in this formulation something akin to Winnicott's famous declaration that 'there is no such thing as a baby'. That is, from a certain perspective, the functioning of the infant – or analysand – cannot be considered outside of its position within the particular and unique facilitating environment provided by its primary caretaker – or analyst. Ferro united these dyadic, intersubjective formulations with the work of the Barangers (Baranger and Baranger, 2009), and elaborated upon the idea that the minds of the analyst and patient together form a Field. The latter defines a conceptual space inside of which whatever occurs to either member of the dyad can be seen as a reflection of and commentary on their relationship and interaction.[10]

The analytic Field

'The Field' is the name we give to the emotional dimension created by the unconscious affective interaction and inter-affectivity of the patient and analyst in the context of the analytic process. Derived from the work of Bion, Merleau-Ponty and Kurt Lewin and introduced into psychoanalysis by Willi and Madeleine Baranger (2009; Baranger et al., 1983), the Field concept has been expanded by Ferro into one of his most fruitful innovations and a powerful clinical tool. This dimension of the analytic process is unique, pair-specific, unconsciously co-constructed and emerges in the analysis as the patient's needs – for affect regulation, growth and development, symptom relief, gratification, coherence and unification of self, etc. – meet the analyst's commitment to participate in a process in which transformations that support the fulfillment of these needs may be realized. It is the uniqueness of analytic relating, with the analyst and patient occupying paradoxical and dialectical roles for each other – presence/absence; reality/fantasy; external/internal; conscious/unconscious – that helps promote the qualities of relationship that allow for the conceptualization and operational assumptions about the existence and nature of the Field.

In clinical terms, the main implication of the existence of the Field is that *the narrative and action of the analytic session, especially as they reflect the emotional disturbances caused by the presence, actions and interventions of the analyst, offer an unconscious running commentary on the quality and condition of the analytic relationship and process, including the patient's experience of the degree of accessibility and availability of the analyst's mind and emotional state.* Thus, from the perspective of the Field, the manifest content of the patient's discourse is to the underlying feeling of the analytic moment as the manifest content of the night dream is to the latent dream thoughts.

> Field theory radically changes how we listen to the patient's communication, which will be seen as also a product of the quality of the analyst's mental functioning or malfunctioning [i.e. the patient's reaction to the analyst's capacities to contain and transform the patient's anxieties and projective identifications]. At the same time, this is also very helpful inasmuch as the patient always functions as a mirror and reflects any movement of the analyst, when s/he comes too close or moves too far away. The analyst will thus be able to make use, among other things, of what the patient signals, to change his or her interpretive attitude.
>
> (Ferro, 2005c, pp. 93–94)

It is for this reason that Bion asserted that the patient is the analyst's best supervisor.

If, for example, I suggest to a patient that my having announced my upcoming vacation seems to be making him upset and he responds with associations about an argumentative boss who must always have the last word in things, I can hear this comment in one of a number of possible ways: as a true piece of external reality; as a piece of transference of the genetic past; as a statement about the patient's internal object world; and so on. Unless we believe the patient is lying, we assume, from the perspective of external reality, the truth of what is being told to us. However, *from the perspective of the Field*, we also assume that that story is unconsciously chosen to be told at this moment, because it efficiently conveys additional levels of meaning that are directly related to and reflective of the analytic relationship and the patient's sense of the analyst's immediate receptivity and activity.

In this sense, each affect and episode in the patient's discourse, like each element of the day residue of the night time dream, is multi-determined and unconsciously chosen to convey an important 'signal from the Field'.[11] As a practical matter of technique, from the Field perspective, each statement that the patient makes or story that the patient tells can be heard as if it were preceded by the introductory phrase, 'last night I had a dream that ...'. The imagined insertion of this phrase may help analysts move beyond the concrete and immediate manifest meanings of what the patient has to say and so soften their focus on the literal, manifest subject and object of the patient's discourse, concentrating instead on its affective quality and/or meaning.

Characters as affective holograms

Ferro captures this aspect of analytic listening in his formulation that, from the perspective of the Field, each character in the patient's narrative may, in addition to its other meanings, be viewed as an 'affective hologram' or emotional constellation independent of the manifest subject or object to which it is attached in the discourse. Another way of describing this perspective is to view the Field as if it were a giant weather map, with each statement implying the possible beginning formation of a new weather disturbance.

In the argumentative boss incident, for example, what may matter most from the Field perspective is that the disturbance introduced by my naming my impending absence as a cause of upset produced a gathering emotional 'weather front' of 'argumentativeness' in the Field. At first, it may neither be necessary nor possible to assign that affect to a subject or object – e.g. neither the actual boss, nor the patient in the transference. (As Pirandello might have said, this 'truth' is still a blur in motion; it is still 'a character in search of an author'.) For instance, it might eventually turn out that what will be most useful is to see the analyst as the one who is 'argumentative'. At this early point in this sequence, it may suffice for the analyst to silently note that a disturbance in the form of 'argumentativeness' has entered the Field. Who it belongs to, how much strength it will gather, what role it may play and so forth will have to be determined by future events.

One of the great challenges of analytic listening is that each of us tends to get diverted from psychic reality by being caught up in the actuality of the patient's story. That we do so is in part a reflection of our everyday assumptions about 'ordinary listening'. When someone in our extra-analytic life tells us a story, we tend to believe it and take it at face value. For example, when a friend tells us about his mother, then we assume that the story is accurate, that the mother in the story we hear today is the same person as the mother that we heard about last week and so on. While the same is true for our patients, *at the same time and from the Field perspective* – or we might say from the perspective of psychic reality rather than literal, historical truth – the identity and continuity of 'the mother' may be highly arbitrary and interchangeable, just as it might be in a night dream, where 'the mother' in the manifest content might represent the analyst, the wife, any other character, real or imagined in the patient's life or thought, a part of the patient's self, etc.

To return to the story of the argumentative boss, the 'message from the field' in that bit of narrative might be that the content of my interpretation was too definitive (i.e. 'saturated') in locking down the meaning of my patient's response or that my being the one to name his affect state might have felt too intrusive, like a 'bossy' imposition. Still another possibility may be that while the content of my 'bossy' interpretation may have been accurate – we must of course also consider the possibility that the patient's response is signaling that my interpretation of the 'bossy analyst' was incorrect! – something might have been amiss in the tact or timing of my interpretation and may have overwhelmed or stirred the patient up excessively. Assuming the latter was the case would not necessarily mean that the interpretation was poorly timed or 'incorrect'. Rather, we must recognize that any and all of our actions and interventions, including that of remaining silent, are apt to produce turbulence in the patient and that that turbulence and the patient's reaction to it, including hints of what the patient may need us to do in order to help them deal with it, is apt to be unconsciously and indirectly reflected in the next set of 'signals from the field' embedded in the analytic process and discourse.

There is sufficient freedom in this process of listening and interpreting to ensure that any presumptive meanings of the messages from the field will be left up to the intuition and creativity of the analyst and patient based in part on what each participant subsequently adds to the co-creation of the analytic discourse and process and in part on what the analyst discerns from his or her subsequent, ongoing attempts to 'read' and interpret the feedback from the field. Thus, as opposed to 'archeological' theories in which the analyst uncovers fixed and hidden facts and meanings,

> Reality in the field is more virtual in nature, involving characters who are progressively subjected to a process of casting in order to express the types of functioning active in the field. All the field's characters are born of mental mating of the two members of the couple, namely the two minds; there is so to speak a continuous summoning up of characters and players, or an ongoing assignment of roles directed towards making the deepest levels of the field more and more susceptible to explicit expression.
>
> (Ferro and Basile, 2009, pp. 2–3)

The Field, then, is a transitional space, which reflects the here-and-now of the analytic situation and a matrix, which provides the primordial substance from which psychic growth and transformation will emerge. Seen from this perspective, the analytic discourse is a Winnicottian Squiggle Game played with inferences, affects and words instead of lines on a paper.

These formulations about the Field allow for the emergence of *a spectrum of possible interpreted meanings* rather than a singular 'truth', each of which will be confirmed, disconfirmed, amended, etc. by the next event that happens or narrative element that is related. This continual feedback process offers potential correctives against wild analysis and the untoward imposition of the analyst's meaning upon the patient's discourse. It also explains why the exact evolution of any given analytic process is so highly dependent in part upon the analyst's subjectivity; it sheds light upon why so many different pathways towards successful analytic work can exist for any given patient depending upon who the analyst is that the patient is paired with and it places the concept of *nachtraglichkeit* (*après coup*) at the center of our understanding of the unfolding of the analytic process.

Unsaturated interpretations and the co-construction of narratives

Assuming the content of my 'boss interpretation' was correct, I would then have three possible categories of response. The first, and perhaps most familiar, is to offer a specific interpretation about what I think may be going on. For example, I could *name the bossy superior in the here-and-now of the transference* – e.g. suggest that the boss association indicates that the patient has responded to my last comment as too bossy and my wanting to have the last word or I could link the patient's presumptive view of me as bossy with old feelings we know existed towards the patient's father or mother, etc. These kinds of interpretations are what Ferro, following Bion, called 'saturated', because their meanings are fixed and fully implied.

A second possibility is that I could *silently read this message from the Field and use the information it contains to recalibrate my listening perspective and the quantity and quality of my interventions*. For instance, I might conclude that it is important at this moment in time for this patient to arrive at his own insights and so, for the time being, hold back from or slow the rate of my making definitive ('saturated') interpretations and see what develops. However, if further signals indicated that the analyst's silence was not proving useful, a third possibility might be to *try to play a somewhat more active, but catalytic and secondary role in the process*.

Were I to take this latter option, I would be in a position analogous to that of a child analyst, who decides at a given moment not to silently observe what his child patient is doing or explicitly interpret the meaning of his child patient's play, but instead joins in and assumes a role within the context of the child's activity or game, aware of certain assumptions that have arisen about what some of the underlying conflicts, fantasies and anxieties are that are being addressed, letting that knowledge inform his moves in the play initiated by the child. This last category of intervention, which will have certain meanings and implications but will still allow room for additional interpretations or developments of meaning, is what Ferro has called an *unsaturated interpretation*.

The recognition that significant work of adult analysis can be carried on by the co-constructive building of narratives, what Ferro (2006) calls 'story-telling', in a fashion that is analogous to play therapy with children is another of Ferro's important contributions and follows from his appreciation of *the plasticity of narrative discourse in relation to the underlying alpha elements from which it is derived.* Whereas in classical analytic formulations, certain narrative themes – e.g. descriptions of relationships with parents and siblings during formative childhood years; overt references to the analytic relationship; derivatives of infantile sexual and aggressive feelings, relationships and conflicts, of Oedipal constellations or conflicts or of the primal scene; etc. – were considered to be bedrock[12] and therefore privileged over others as the 'true north' of analytic investigation, Ferro has argued that from the perspective of the Field, each of these or any other narrative content in the patient's discourse may be viewed as equally relevant and interchangeable, because their main function as signals from the Field is to comment on the emotions emerging and in need of containment, metabolization and transformation in patient, analyst and the analytic relationship and situation of the moment.

Alpha elements, narrative dialects and the plasticity of narrative

As we have noted above, except in those infrequent instances when they occur as visual 'flashes', alpha elements are rarely noticed or experienced in their pure form. They can, however, be inferred by the narrative derivative sequences to which they give rise. Ferro (2002a, 2005a, 2005b) has written about this at length, offering many illustrations of how a unique series of alpha elements may underlie, give rise to and be expressed by different 'narrative dialects'. For example, he (Ferro, 2005b) offers the following hypothetical illustration in which the analyst's interpretation produces great distress (turbulence), causing the patient to feel proto-emotions (so called, because they are not yet formed and so are barely discernible and comprehensible), which we might label as pain, anger and revenge. In his illustration, these beta elements lead to the formation of the following hypothetical alpha elements:

A CHILD WHO CRIES (pain)
A HURRICANE (anger)
A MAN WHO FIRES A GUN (revenge)

These alpha elements would only be known indirectly, by inference, through the potential derivative narrative sequences in the patient's discourse to which they give rise. Some of the different possible narrative derivatives that could be built around these alpha elements would be constructed from different 'dialects', each of which would convey the same emotional sequence, but in different words (e.g. the 'language' of childhood memory; the 'language' of a movie one had recently seen; 'the language' of a night dream; etc.).

For example, the above sequence might be conveyed:

- *Through a childhood memory*: 'I remember the hurt the doctor caused when he took out my tonsils, the fury I felt and how I slapped him as soon as my hands were free'. Or, 'I remember the schoolyard fight in which a bully beat me up. I was so angry that I slashed his bicycle tires!'
- *Through external events*: 'I saw a news story of a boy whose dog was hit by a motorist. The boy became enraged, chased the car down and beat up the driver'.
- *Through a sexual episode*: 'My boyfriend was so brutal and insensitive in forcing me to have sex with him that I refused to speak to him for a week and tore up all the photos of our trip'.

(Ferro, 2005b, pp. 425–426)

The analyst who hears any of these descriptions must be able to consider them from multiple perspectives: e.g. as true descriptions of external reality; as symbolic references to the genetic past; as a symbolic description of the patient's current, internal object world; etc. But from the perspective of the Field, the patient's narrative may be viewed as a kind of 'analytic GPS signal', or commentary upon the analytic situation that will allow the analyst to make an inference about how the patient is experiencing what is going on between them and what the patient needs.

To the extent that the patient is always talking about something and that that 'something' is always functioning as an analytic GPS signal and that the analyst is always taking account of and responding to that signal and the patient is offering further commentary, etc., then the analytic dialogue may be seen as an ongoing, self-regulating Squiggle Game taking place between adults, in which words are used as the 'squiggles' that interact playfully in helping an image, thought feeling or narrative clarify, sharpen and/or emerge from unconsciousness or come into being for the first time.

Ferro's interest in storytelling and the creation of narratives has led him to recognize that the analyst has a wide range of possibilities ('analyst's squiggles') beyond those of interpretation or inquiry at his or her disposal in response to the patient's discourse ('patient squiggles'). In general, he describes the analyst's interventions in terms of the degree to which they are 'saturated' (relatively specific and fixed in meaning, e.g. 'you are angry at me now, because you feel that I am trying to restrict your choice and freedom, like your father did when you were in High School and he forbade you to date Martina, because she was of a different religion and social class') or 'unsaturated' (ambiguous, framed within the 'dialect' of the patient's manifest content and open to various meanings and interpretations, e.g. 'nobody likes being pushed around and told what to do and that can certainly stir up a lot of feelings').

The distinction in the options of the analyst's interventions that Ferro is making here, between saturated and unsaturated interpretations, is analogous to the difference between *interpretations of the transference* and *interpretations from within the transference*, which has been described in French psycho-analysis (Sechaud, 2008). What the Squiggle Game/child analysis perspective adds to the French formulation, however, is the important possibility that the analyst intervening in the unsaturated mode may do so in a way that his or her intervention will play a 'double role'. That is, from within the perspective of the patient's chosen dialect, the analyst's remarks may appear to be a comment in keeping with the manifest content that continues the discourse in a derivative and displaced fashion. Within the privacy of the analyst's own mind, however, the comment may be framed so as also to stand in as an inferred comment about the transference. Thus, if I were to reply to my patient in an unsaturated fashion that a boss who responded like that might make someone furious, I would not only be talking to the patient about the ostensible or reported reality of his work situation, I would also be taking the 'character' 'furious' out of our hypothetical toy box and offering it a place in our play, while noting in my mind that perhaps the fury I was referring to was building inside my patient towards me for having mentioned my impending absence or having made the interpretation that 'decided' or announced the 'reality' of what he presumably was feeling.

The value to the analyst of having a theory that keeps open a channel for expecting communications from the Field is that whatever level of response is offered by the patient or inferred by the analyst, its accuracy or usefulness will be immediately indicated by further feedback embedded in the patient's next response. Consistently following these 'messages from the Field' allows us to better describe *the choreography of change* within the analysis in which process and non-process, movement and impasse, combine and resolve, only to recur in new manifestations, in a never-ending dialectic. This dialectic describes a two-person 'dance', in which symbolic repetitions of traumatic and conflicted situations and relationships are unconsciously actualized within the analytic couple (enactments), recognized by one or another of the pair and analyzed or otherwise transformed – 'corrected', so to speak – so that micro-impasses emerge, are recognized and addressed and then give way to developmentally progressive process.

This formulation reflects another of Ferro's (2002a, 2005b) important ela-borations of Bion's work: his recognition that insight is neither an end in itself nor is it the only possible means to the end of catalyzing and producing change (transformations). In classical formulations, where repression pro-duces resistance, which yields to interpretation and gives rise to remembering the forgotten past, insight and its subsequent working through, is the agent par excellence of transformation. As such, insight (i.e. *content*) is apt to be seen as the end rather than the means of therapeutic action.

In contrast, Ferro's description of micro-transformations through the facil-itation of development of the patient's narratives as an important therapeutic factor reminds us *that the therapeutic end of analytic treatment lies in process (transformation and psychic growth), no matter how it is catalyzed or arrived at.*

Thus, it is as important to read the constant feedback signals from the Field in order to adjust the analyst's internal listening stance and degree of responsiveness and/or to anticipate the kind of unsaturated contribution that will offer the next step in the co-construction of the patient's narrative, as it is to use them to formulate decoding transference interpretations of how the patient is experiencing the analysis and analytic relationship in the here-and-now or in the light of past relationships.

Conclusions

At the heart of Ferro's work is a vision of the analytic process that is transformational in its aims and intersubjective in its means. For Ferro, as for Bion, the ultimate aim of psychoanalysis is the creation of thought and the creation of mind.

> The aim of the analysis is to develop the patient's ability to 'dream' – and hence, to transform, metabolize and therefore forget – the excesses of sensoriality and proto-emotions which, unless digested and 'dreamed', lead to suffering and symptoms.
>
> (Ferro and Basile, 2009, p. 11)

The mental functioning and activity of the analyst plays a major catalytic role in this creative process and is a central co-determinant of the analytic Field. The latter is an unconscious and inevitable co-construction of the analytic dyad that is made up of contributions from each member, but is more than the sum of its parts. It is the product and location of the emotional turbulence activated by the analytic encounter and it is the locus and matrix for the transformational processes of the analytic cure. Through his adumbration and elaboration of Field Theory, Ferro

> changes the paradigm of analytic work from the unveiling of a hidden meaning to facilitating the possibility of [the patient's] thinking for oneself of possible new meanings. The psychoanalytic laboratory then becomes dedicated not to what has been but to what may be in the future.
>
> (Ferro and Basile, 2009, p. 3)

Notes

1 Portions of this chapter previously appeared in Levine, H.B. (2015). The transformational vision of Antonino Ferro. *Psychoanalytic Inquiry*, 35: 451–464. We gratefully acknowledge their permission to expand upon and reprint this material.
2 'Psychoanalysis is not a symbolic system charged with "deciphering meaning", but a "system for generating new thoughts"' (Ferro, 2006, p. 92).
3 Quoted in Ferro (2005b, p. 61).

4 Bion offers analysts a model of the mind and 'instruments with which we can think without telling us *what* to think' (Ferro, 2005b, p. 424).

5 As we shall see below, Ferro made a major contribution when he recognized that there was a perspective from which *all* of the patient's past historical and extra-analytic descriptions could be seen as a running unconscious commentary on the immediate, subjective, emotional experience of the analytic session and therefore could be heard as an aspect of the here-and-now.

6

> ... dreaming is a constant activity carried out by our psychic apparatus, even when we are awake. This means that the mental work of wakefulness consists of forming images that sum up, just as in night dreams, the emotional quality of what we are living at that moment. What we 'say' is the narrative derivative of these images.
>
> (Ferro, 2005b, p. 429)

7 In this sense, beta elements are reminiscent of Freud's (1915a) description of the drives as a 'frontier concept' between psyche and soma.

8 See also Rocha Barros (2000).

9 Bion often writes the words 'represent' and 'representation', with a hyphen between the 're' and the 'p' to indicate the dialectical tension and relationship that exist between the analyst's absorption and metabolization of the patient's undigested beta elements, the return ('re-presentation)' of the now transformed once beta now alpha elements (i.e. once intolerable now made tolerable) to the patient and the patient's newly enhanced or created capacity for psychic representation that may emerge in this process.

10 'Together, patient and analyst structure a field that is a function of the inner lives of both participants, brought together by a shared basic unconscious phantasy, which develops at that very moment when the setting is constituted' (Ferro, 2005c, p. 88).

11 The same is true for each of the patient's actions that are precipitated by the analysis. I have chosen here to emphasize the patient's discourse, because I believe that analysts are less comfortable assuming the fungibility of characters in the patient's discourse than they are reading unconscious meaning into enactments and other forms of patient behavior.

12 Recall that in 'Analysis terminable and interminable', Freud (1937) said that the castration complex in women and passivity in men were the 'bedrocks' of analytic work beyond which psychoanalysis could not penetrate.

References

Baranger, W. and Baranger, M. (2009). *The Work of Confluence: Listening and Interpreting in the Psychoanalytic Field*. Ed. by L.G. Fiorini. London: Karnac.

Baranger, W., Baranger, M. and Mom, J. (1983). Process and non-process in analytic work. *International Journal of Psychoanalysis*, 64: 1–16.

Bion, W.R. (1962a). The psycho-analytic study of thinking. *International Journal of Psychoanalysis*, 43: 306–310.

Bion, W.R. (1962b). *Learning From Experience*. London: Heinemann.

Bion, W.R. (1970). *Attention and Interpretation*. London: Heinemann.

Bion, W.R. (2005). *The Italian Seminars*. London: Karnac.

Botella, C. and Botella, S. (2005). *The Work of Psychic Figurability*. Abingdon: Routledge.

Ferro, A. (2002a). *In The Analyst's Consulting Room*. London: Routledge.

Ferro, A. (2002b). Some implications of Bion's thought. *International Journal of Psychoanalysis*, 83: 597–608.

Ferro, A. (2005a). Which reality in the psychoanalytic session? *Psychoanalysis Quarterly*, 74: 421–442.

Ferro, A. (2005b). *Seeds of Illness, Seeds of Recovery: The Genesis of Suffering and the Role of Psychoanalysis*. Trans. by P. Slotkin. Hove and New York: Brunner-Routledge.

Ferro, A. (2005c). Commentary on Field Theory by Madeleine Baranger. In *Truth, Reality and The Psychoanalyst*. Ed. by S. Lewkowicz and S. Flechner. London: IPA. pp. 87–96.

Ferro, A. (2006). *Psychoanalysis as Therapy and Storytelling*. Hove and New York: Routledge.

Ferro, A. and Basile, R. (Eds) (2009). *The Analytic Field: A Clinical Concept*. London: Karnac.

Freud, S. (1911). *Formulations on the two principles of mental functioning*. S.E. 12, pp. 213–226.

Freud, S. (1915a). *Instincts and their vicissitudes*. S.E. 14, pp. 109–140.

Freud, S. (1915b). *The unconscious*. S.E. 14, pp. 159–216.

Freud, S. (1923). *The Ego and the Id*. S.E. 19, pp. 3–68.

Freud, S. (1933). *New introductory lectures on psycho-analysis*. S.E. 22, pp. 3–184.

Freud, S. (1937). *Analysis terminable and interminable*. S.E. 23, pp. 209–254.

Levine, H.B. (2006). Book Review: *Seeds of Illness, Seeds of Recovery: The Genesis of Suffering and the Role of Psychoanalysis*. By Antonino Ferro. Trans. by Philip Slotkin. *Journal of the American Psychoanalytic Association*, 54: 670–677.

Ogden, T. (1994). The analytic third: Working with intersubjective clinical facts. *International Journal of Psychoanalysis*, 75: 3–20.

Parisi, M. (2009). The use of alpha function in analytical construction. Paper given at the International Psychoanalytic Association Congress, Chicago, July.

Rocha Barros, E. (2000). Affect and pictographic image: The constitution of meaning in mental life. *International Journal of Psychoanalysis*, 81: 1087–1099.

Sechaud, E. (2008). The handling of the transference in French psychoanalysis. *International Journal of Psychoanalysis*, 89: 1011–1028.

Spillius, E.B. (1992). Clinical experiences of projective identification. In *Clinical Lectures on Bion and Klein*. Ed. by R. Anderson. London: Routledge, pp 59–73.

Chapter 2

The logic of the Field[1,2]

Howard B. Levine

The Field is a concept that, with a few exceptions, is newly arrived in Anglophone psychoanalysis, mostly by way of Antonino Ferro's (e.g. 2002, 2005, 2006) application of the work of Bion, Winnicott and the Barangers.[3] Its many antecedents include the Gestalt theory of Kurt Lewin and the phenomenology of Merleau-Ponty. Its psychoanalytic roots, firmly planted in the work of Willy and Madeleine Baranger (e.g. 2008, 2009), extend back as far as Freud's (1912, p. 115) declaration that the unconscious of one person may be in direct contact with the unconscious of another; Bion's (1961) observation that groups behave as if they possessed a shared, primordial unconscious and the formulation of the communicative dimension of projective identification, alpha function and container/contained (Bion 1962, 1970); Joseph's (1985) adumbration of Klein's 'total situation transference'; and the many contributors to the recognition and articulation of the intersubjective dimension of the psychoanalytic encounter.[4] Among Anglophone analysts, however, the definition and technical implications of the Field have not been well established, nor substantively agreed upon.[5]

The nature of the Field is such that its contents and form cannot be fully specifiable. They are inherently *emergent*. The Field is a concept that – and this is its strength and value – exults in the domain of the unsaturated, always becoming, and is never complete on its own, in that its very nature is that, although at each moment it reflects and comments upon what has gone before, it also asks to be completed by a contribution from the subjectivity of the other. How then to define or describe it? Is it the Bionian Field? The Ferro-ian Field? The Field of the Barangers? Or will what I hope to describe, by necessity, be redolent of my own subjectivity?

In the essay that follows, I will attempt to articulate my sense of its meaning and potential value in the clinical encounter and add a brief clinical illustration in the hopes that this may be found useful by others.

What do we mean by the psychoanalytic Field?

The psychoanalytic situation is a two-person, intersubjective encounter constituted by the patient, the analyst, the setting and the method. 'The Field' is

DOI: 10.4324/9781003168034-2

the name we give to the *hypothesis* that there is an emotional dimension created by the conscious and unconscious affective interaction and inter-affectivity of the patient and analyst in the context of the analytic process that is greater than the sum of its constituent parts. This dimension is unique, pair-specific, unconsciously co-constructed and emerges in the analysis as the patient's needs – for affect regulation, growth and development, symptom relief, gratification, coherence and unification of self, etc. – meet the analyst's ethical commitment (Chetrit-Vatine, 2004) to participate in a process in which transformations that will support the fulfillment of these needs may be realized.

As I have come to understand and use the concept, it has important implications for analytic listening, for monitoring the degrees of freedom available moment-to-moment in the analytic process and for establishing a presumptive feedback system of unconscious commentary on that process and how it is being experienced by the patient in the here-and-now. The latter offers the analyst a way of tentatively assessing and optimizing the rhythm, strength, frequency and degree of saturation of interpretations and the accessibility of the patient to interpretations *in* or *of* the transference.[6]

It is the uniqueness of analytic relating, with the analyst and patient occupying paradoxical, enigmatic and dialectical roles for each other – presence/absence; reality/fantasy; external/internal; conscious/unconscious; found/created – that helps promote the qualities of relationship that allow for the conceptualization and operational assumptions about the existence and nature of the Field. While there is a certain asymmetry of purpose and intent within the distribution of these roles, in that the predominant direction of the gradient container/contained moves from patient (projector) to analyst (recipient), there is also a degree, no matter how small, to which the gradient may be reversed and the patient may function as a container for the projections of the analyst. However, I believe that in a well-functioning, 'good enough' analysis – i.e. barring major countertransference interferences – the latter present a minor, although always significant contribution, and may always be present.

When this reversal of gradient does appear, its presence should prompt analytic reflection and/or exploration. This exploration may be silent on the analyst's part or made part of the manifest discourse, depending on the specific circumstances. It is important to be aware that at times this reversal of projective gradient may represent an unconscious actualization of a negative transference object that is being 'cast' and brought forward into the aliveness of the analytic situation.

To the extent that reverse projective identification is present, it also raises questions about whether or to what extent its working through may become 'curative' for the analyst. Will such a serendipitous analytic result prove detrimental to the development of the patient? The answer will be specific to each analytic moment and encounter and its appropriateness must be evaluated in the ethical context of the *patient's* clinical and developmental needs.

The truth status of the Field

I emphasize that *the Field is a hypothesis*, because it is an abstract concept in danger of becoming reified. Whether such a thing as the Field actually 'exists' in concrete reality or is simply a pragmatic assumption that assists the analyst in his or her clinical task is a moot point. The Field is an aspect of *psychic reality* and as such, its status in veridical reality may well be immaterial in comparison to its pragmatic use in the clinical setting.

The pursuit and understanding of the psychoanalytic object, psychic reality and the unconscious require a psychoanalytically informed intuition that is something more than simple empirical observation. Bion (1970) argued that emotional reality and states of mind are not amenable to direct observation by the senses and that their detection must rest upon intuition rather than empirical observation. This of course opens us up to the danger of tendentious and countertransference-driven false intuitions.

In his Tavistock Seminars, Bion (2005) considered this possibility when he wrote:

> When we are at a loss we invent something to fill the gap of our ignorance ... The more frightening the gap ... the more we are pressed from outside and inside to fill the gap ...
>
> [I]n a situation where you feel completely lost ... you are thankful to clutch hold of any system, anything whatever that is available on which to build a kind of structure. So from this point of view it seems to me that we could argue that the whole of psychoanalysis fills a long-felt want by being a vast Dionysiac system; since we don't know what is there, we invent these theories and build this glorious structure that has no foundation in fact – or the only fact in which it has any foundation is our complete ignorance, our lack of capacity.
>
> (p. 2)

The saving grace is that this is not always and inevitably the case: 'However, we hope ... that psychoanalytic theories [and interpretations] would remind you of real life at some point in the same way as a good novel or a good play would remind you how human beings behave' (ibid.).

Thus, it is incidental whether or not propositions in psychoanalysis and its metapsychology turn out to be demonstrable or proven in 'real world' terms or are verified or supported by the findings of other disciplines. Psychoanalysis as a clinical praxis, at certain points and perhaps even in large measure, rests upon a theory of psychic functioning and therapeutic action that, in 'reminding us how human beings behave', may answer only to the questions: 'Is it clinically useful to make this assumption? And if so, how?'

The epistemology of the Field

The domain of psychic reality is the realm of the ineffable (Bion, 1970). There are major epistemological differences between psychic reality and consensually validatable social or 'commonsense' reality and these spill over into our psychoanalytic usage and understanding of what we mean by the Field and 'the unconscious' and extend to related concepts such as 'memory', 'thought' and 'perception'.[7]

When viewed from the perspective of everyday life, the epistemology of the Field is counterintuitive. Its logic is that of psychic reality and transitional space, rather than consensually validatable social reality. To put it another way, we live in a quantum universe (where the hard truth of veridical reality is incomplete, unknowable and even to some degree fungible[8]), but, in most situations, in order to negotiate the socially shared (seeming) 'reality' of our everyday lives, we operate as if we lived in a Newtonian space.

Similarly, in psychic reality and the realm of the unconscious, time is not linear, but syncretic rather than diachronic; time's arrow is reversible (think here of *après coup*) and in regard to the unrepresented and emergent, what Scarfone (2006) has called 'the unpast', past and future are enigmatic, fluid and yet to be determined.

Bion (1970) addressed an important dimension of this epistemological divide in *Attention and Interpretation*, when he said that psychoanalytic inquiry is dependent upon the recognition and exploration of a kind of experience that is not of the senses. While a physician may observe (see) a patient's jaundice, feel (touch) their irregular pulse, or recoil at the stench (smell) of an infected wound, 'the realizations with which a psycho-analyst deals cannot be seen or touched; anxiety has no shape or colour, smell or sound' (p. 7).

Of course, anxiety may produce physiological changes that are observable, such as rapid pulse or respirations, sweating, etc. However, Bion considered these to be secondary to the thing-in-itself, the psychic state. While they may lead one to infer its presence, that inference or indication is not assumed to be the same as observing the psychic state.

If Bion is correct, then he is in a sense – or in some instances – questioning the value of empirical observation as a fundamental tool for psychoanalysis. It is for this reason that he proposed 'the term "intuit" as a parallel in the psychoanalyst's domain to the physician's use of "see", "touch", "smell", and "hear"' (Bion, 1970, p. 7). In elevating the analyst's intuition to a place analogous to that of empirical observation in physical medicine, Bion was implicitly indicating that *the realm of psychic reality, 'the psychoanalytic object', is the ultimate locus of psychoanalytic investigation and concern.*

The nature of experience

According to the logic of the Field, every comment and psychic occurrence (feeling, thought, phantasy, action, impulse, defense, etc.) within or between either participant can be assumed to have an unconscious, intersubjective, communicative dimension that reflects the affective forces operating within and between the dyad at each moment, and so is a phenomenon of the Field. The analytic situation offers us a 'thick slide' of experience under the 'analytic microscope' and as we minutely focus up and down, we may bring into focus the intrapsychic, the interpersonal, the object relational, the transferential, etc. perspective of each participant or the perspective of the Field. Where we settle at any given moment is a function of the vertex of our observation.

In the preceding paragraph, I have spoken, quite colloquially, of 'experience', but this term, too, needs further explication. We must ask what we mean by Experience. Following Bion's (1962, 1970) distinction between O (raw existential Experience) and K (that part of Experience that one can come to know and specify in words), I (Levine, 2010, 2015b) have proposed using the convention of distinguishing between 'capital E Experience' (O) and 'small e experience' (K, that part of Experience that can become known)', accepting Bion's view that Experience (O) itself is never fully knowable. Only parts of that Experience may come into the domain of that which can be known (K) and become part of our 'small e' experience.

This means that *transformations from O to K (T(O)→K) are not necessarily fixed one-to-one correspondences and never move from a fully saturated element in one domain to a fully saturated element in another. Whether we are speaking of perception, memory, somatic sensation, drive feeling or other psychic qualities, there is always some enigmatic, ambiguous, not-yet-completed ideational form that is emergent and context-specific.* In analysis, the context is the pair within the setting. The nature of lived experience is such that *the human organism registers experience, internal and external, drive and perception, as vague somatic sensations.* These must be transformed – 'dreamed' in Bion's (1962, 1970, 1992) terms – to be given meaning and made personally meaningful, 'subjectivized', 'personalized' and instantiated into a fixed temporal sequence.

Another way of describing this is to say that each stimulus – internal or external, drive, somatic sensation or perception – produces an affect or sensation that then needs to find a suitable container. In general, there are several different categories of container for affect. These include words (in the form of ideas, names of categories, symbols and metaphors), actions, aesthetic forms (music, plastic arts, etc.) and feelings.

Discussing this phenomenon in relation to the psychic representation of the drives and the consequences of pre-verbal trauma to one's sense of self, Roussillon (2011) notes that

> the languages of the act and body remain in effect fundamentally ambiguous. They bear a potential, virtual meaning, but one that depends on the meaning that the object, to which it is directed, gives to it. It is a language which … must 'be interpreted'. It is but the potential for meaning, the bearer of potential: it is meaning that has not yet been

finished ... It seeks a respondent, it does not exhaust its meaning in a single expression, and the reaction or the response of the object is necessary for its signifying integration ... [W]hen the respondent has not been located or has not given an adequate subjectifying reply, the potential meaning loses its generative power.

(pp. 203–204)

For purposes of clarity, I am proposing that we use the terms 'affect' and 'feeling' in a way that is not equivalent or interchangeable. *Affect* will refer to something that is 'somatic' (*actual* and of the body; proto- or pre-psychic and not yet psychically represented; a part of O that has not yet been transformed into K). *Feeling* is psychic and represented. It is the part of O that is knowable or has become known via the work of psychic transformation, which Bion (1965) denoted as T(O)→K. However, even though feeling is represented, it is never fully saturated or defined. Like affect and action, as communication or 'dialect' of discourse, feeling always contains a dimension that is enigmatic, ambiguous and therefore to some extent unsaturated and emergent, awaiting completion by the response of or interaction with the other.

Transforming experience/creating experience

In order for T(O)→K, for Experience→experience, something ineffable must be transformed, and this requires a suitable container. The suitable containers for Experience – what can capture, transform and give shape, content and meaning to raw affect – are aesthetic, metaphoric and symbolic forms,[9] ideas, feelings and actions. The latter two may carry or convey 'meaning' only in the semiotic[10] sense. Their meaning is not as saturated as meanings conveyed by more semantic (i.e. word-based) elements. Hence, their nature is often more ambiguous, enigmatic and not yet fully completed or emerged. They await completion by the participation, contribution and transformational action of an other-subject, which not only must receive, recognize and respond to the signal as communication (Roussillon, 2011), but must help transform it into something knowable or at least tolerable (Bion, 1962, 1970). (The reduction of tension in making something tolerable allows room for knowing, even if it is only a clearing of the mind so that one can come to know something else!)

In Ferro's work (e.g. 2002, 2005, 2006), there are many examples in which a series of not yet mentalized sensorial disturbances (beta elements) are transformed into possible narrative 'dialects' – e.g. the dialect of a description of an encounter with a boyfriend, a memory from childhood, an association to an episode in a movie that the patient has just heard about, a dream from last night, etc. The metaphors that I use to try to characterize and think about this dimension of the Field are that of the Pirandello (1998) play *Six Characters in Search of an Author*, where the characters plead to be put into a storyline that will allow them to achieve a meaningful context, and the story of the hermit crab. The latter is a creature that lives at the seashore, but cannot secrete a shell of its own. Instead, it adapts itself to whatever potential carapace it finds along its way and adopts that as its shell or house. Thus, it can use as its 'shell' the discarded fragment of a lobster or mollusk shell, a bit of cardboard, plastic or wood, and so on. In the same way, pre-psychic sensorial disturbances (beta elements; affect) can 'find a home' and a narrative discourse in any number of possible bits of stories ('narremes').

I think that Bion (1963) intuited something of this when he wrote that interpretations would be more effective if they included extensions in the domain of myth. Adding a narrative, metaphoric dimension to an interpretation is a way of challenging or making a demand upon the patient's mind for psychic work, as the ambiguity and polysemic potential of the metaphor acts as an optimally disturbing presence that continues to gnaw and work away through enigmatic means until some resolution and partial completion via working through is achieved.[11] Metaphor (or myth) is also the way that we 'capture' elements of unconscious experience so that they may be 'seen' and reflected upon (Ogden, 1997).

The shadow of the object

The foundations for this line of thinking were already present in Freud. In Mourning and Melancholia, Freud (1917b) famously described how in cases of acute object loss, 'the shadow of the object falls upon the ego'. More broadly, I believe that Freud implicated this principle in all normal development when he declared that the ego was a precipitate of abandoned object relations (Freud, 1917a, 1923). Earlier still, in his 'Screen memories' paper, Freud (1899) suggested that memories were not pristine and stored fully formed, but remained partly unsaturated until recollected and their ultimate specific form was dependent upon the context in which they were retrieved. That is, he implied that their ideational form was completed in the present at the moment of recall and assembled with a specific unconscious purpose in mind.

It is from this deeply Freudian perspective that Roussillon (2011), who finds neuro-scientific confirmation of this position in the work of Gerald Edelman (1989), argues persuasively that 'Development and gradual integration are not automatic or dependent solely on the self's internal processes; they become structured only when they are accompanied by an appropriate response from ... [one's primary] objects' (p. 180).

The self that emerges is then '*constructed in accordance with the nature and type of adjustment and mirroring that the primary object proposes*' (p. 139, italics added). This dependence on the other for discovery of the self is what Roussillon (2011) calls

> the paradox of primary narcissism: cathexis of the object is superposed on that of the self, with no antagonism as long as the cathexis of the object

reflects back to the self its own states of feeling, not necessarily in the same mode.

(pp. 139–140, italics added)

Thus, for Roussillon, the primary object is inevitably a *'symbolizing object'*, one that 'subjectifies the self or enables the self to take on board the feeling of being a subject' (ibid., p. 171). It is this dimension of psychic development that is repeated in the analytic process, charts an important element of its therapeutic action and is central to the creation of and assumptions about the Field:

> The treatment setting ... becomes the arena of an intersubjective relationship in which the interplay between the transference and countertransference becomes a decisive factor. *The shadow of the psychoanalyst falls on the analytic process and treatment*, as it were, *and, with it, the shadow of all the objects that have contributed historically to constructing the self's mental apparatus.*
>
> (ibid., p. 52, italics added)

It is for this reason that construction and attention to the here-and-now of the total transference situation assume such importance in the cure:

> The here-and-now of the psychoanalytic dialogue is the focus of the analyst's attention and lies at the very heart of how the transference is seen; the analysand's actual past has, thus, only a secondary role to play – since meaning is not already there, it has to be constructed in the here-and-now of the analytical process.
>
> (ibid., p. 54)

And it is what describes the relevance and explains the effectiveness of technical and therapeutic assumptions about the Field.

The Field as 'weather map' and 'analytic GPS'

One of the great conundrums of psychoanalytic praxis – and opportunities of the method – is why, at any given moment, a patient chooses to say one thing rather than another. Freud thought that the answer lay in the push for discharge and gratification that was inherent in repressed sexual and aggressive wishes. He later enlarged his view to include defensive motivations and the narcissistic need to repeat and work through elements of traumatic past experience to a better conclusion. To these, I would add – or perhaps restate in a more general and inclusive form – the view, following Bion, Green and others, that the psychic apparatus attempts to deal with not yet mentalized sensorial disturbances – i.e. the disturbance of that which is unrepresented or not yet dreamt and made psychic – by acts of figurability (Botella and Botella, 2005) and other kinds of psychic representation and elaboration.[12]

For the patient, the emotional engagement with and presence of the analyst presents a potentially disturbing and ever-changing, ever-present demand upon the patient's mind for work. The same may also be said for the analyst's mind in regard to the patient. Hence Bion's assertion that in an analysis there ought to be *two* frightened people in the room. However, by virtue of the analyst's personal analysis and training, one would hope that the analyst would be at least a little less frightened and better able to rely upon his or her own capacities for containment, affect tolerance, self-regulation and transformation via representation of affective turbulence.

What this doubly disturbing situation means from the perspective of the Field is that each response coming from each member of the dyad will contain within it and reflect, moment-to-moment, affects related to the shadow of the other and therefore reflect or relate in some way to the emotional quality of their engagement. This is the context in which memories will be formed; the direction in which associations will be primed; the 'grain of sand' that the psyche of each participant will be responding to in a never ending need to resolve the disturbance of emotional contact with oneself and the other by creating the 'pearl' of their personal stream of consciousness and hence constructing the analytic discourse.

This interaffectivity furnishes the rationale for Ferro's (2002, 2005, 2006) assertion that each person and emotional disposition that appears in the manifest or latent discourse of either party can be assumed to represent a 'character' or 'affective hologram' of some emotional disposition that is 'brewing' in the Field. Like the weather fronts on the meteorologist's map, some of these will dissipate and disappear, while others will gather force and grow into more recognizable disturbances or even full-fledged storms. It should be noted that 'characters' in the Field may be *individuals* that appear in the discourse or in phantasy of either participant or may be *emotional qualities or dispositions*, such as 'submission' or 'watchfulness', 'anger' or 'joy'. (Grotstein (2009) has likened their appearance in this form, rather than as 'people', such as 'my uncle Joe' or 'my girlfriend, Sally', etc. to the personification of emotional attitudes – Wisdom, Courage, Greed, etc. – found in medieval Morality Plays).

With this as background, we can better understand the rationale for the assumption that every character – comment, action, feeling, phantasy, etc. – that appears within and between the members of the analytic dyad has a *potential signaling function* that reflects and comments upon what has just transpired between the two. There is thus a perspective from which every story told or imagined, no matter what its truth value, relevance or other meanings might be, is a covert, unconscious reaction to and commentary upon the events and emotions stirred by whatever has just transpired.

Of course, the embedded meaning, the 'signal from the Field', is not always simple, straightforward or easily discernible. But if the analyst listens as Bion (1967, 1970) suggests, without memory, desire or understanding, and lets the experience of being with the patient wash over him or her, stirring and eliciting whatever it might, then there is a chance that a selected fact will appear in the form of a 'signal from the Field' giving presumptive order and meaning to what is transpiring within and/or between them.

The analytic process: Circulation and the Field

The final point I wish to make concerns the analytic process and the change in orientation in analysis from a more or less predominant emphasis on the translation, uncovering or discovering of unconscious, hidden content to including helping the patient develop the tools with which to think. The origins of this shift, which is a veritable sea change in our understanding, goes back at least to Freud's (1937, pp. 262–265). 'Constructions' paper, where he makes what is in retrospect an extraordinary observation that the measure of the accuracy of an analyst's interpretation is not to be found in the manifest acceptance or rejection of that interpretation by the patient, but in the freeing up of the patient's associative process.[13]

Circulation is one of the key dimensions of the Field. To what extent are affects and ideas free to circulate? This is akin, from another vertex or perspective, of asking to what extent the associations of the patient or analyst are truly free. Indeed, Roussillon (2011) has suggested that constriction of associations, i.e. limitation of circulation, is a hallmark of stasis produced by neurotic defense, trauma, countertransference or unconscious collusion. In the terms of the Barangers, such a constriction represents an unconscious collusion or *bastion* and becomes an expression of the 'psychopathology' of the Field.

In regard to the mind of the patient, freedom of circulation includes and follows from the unique and creative expression of associational linkages and the surprise emergence of issues and affects in the manifest discourse. In the analyst, indications of freedom of circulation include the degree of spontaneous internal associational response to the patient's discourse and the rapidity of fluctuations between the appearance and dissolving of selected facts in the mind of the analyst in the oscillation PS↔D. To be lodged in a given vertex for too long presents the probability or at least the danger that a selected fact has become an overvalued idea; that memory or desire has too strongly 'infected' the analyst's analytic functioning.

The latter point about circulation is another way of placing a premium on *negative capability*. An important expectation in analytic listening is that we will come to see new relationships between familiar elements, so that new configurations can appear and have their moment upon the stage. In order to do this, we must tolerate uncertainty and not knowing, as we work through the 'micro-illnesses' that appear in the Field and clamor for attention. When successfully addressed, these will stop recurring in the perseverative way that they tend to unless or until they are worked through and cleared away. In effect, in an analysis that is going well, there is a 'respiration' or 'choreography' of alternating freedoms and constrictions, of knowing and not knowing, of organization, disorganization and re-organization that is a necessary and valorized movement within the process.

From the perspective of 'circulation', transference resistances, negative transferences, undreamt dreams or interrupted dreams, etc. are all 'stuck points' in the free associational circulation of ideas and affects; areas of frozen linkage or de-linkage. Co-construction of narrative may put these back into play. But this is a building or re-building of psychic capacity, an overcoming or working through of defenses, that takes place not necessarily or not only through semantic means (interpretation). It also occurs semiotically via 'play work' with affects and actions, where words may not only convey meaning, but function as actions in a verbal Squiggle Game (Winnicott, 1971).

What circulation and the analyst's action (verbal and otherwise) do is give elements the chance to line up or be seen to be lined up in new configurations. This is the effect of the analyst's enigmatic presence, opening up a space that the patient may then fill in (Laplanche's 'hollowed out transference' or *transference en creux*).[14] It is the 'cue ball effect' of the analyst's words-as-actions that 'break up the rack', as in a pocket billiards game, scattering the balls upon the table into new and different positions and configurations.

In the latter sense, every interpretation, no matter how word-based, content-filled, 'cognitive', 'rational' or 'linear' and redolent of K is also an action and therefore part of and productive of the O of this moment leading to the next. It is an action that reflects and precipitates affect and has the potential to put the elements of the Field (affects, ideas and actions) into motion and circulation. This circulation produces the latest GPS readings that are 'signals from the Field' for the analyst to try to read (intuit and conjecture). Analysts, then, should inevitably expect to find themselves in the position of the character in the cartoon *Pogo*, who could write but couldn't read and so had to depend upon others to read back to him what he had just written. We may consciously know what we intended to say to the patient, but what we did or said or how or what the patient took what we said to mean can only come back to us in the next moment of the Field via the GPS ...

Thus, novelty and surprise are presumptive indicators of process and growth as opposed to stasis and repetition.[15] An exception to this point is that the emergence of stasis in an otherwise 'good enough' analysis may represent progress in the form of the necessary and inevitable actualization of a negative transference object as a character in or a 'micro-illness' of the Field. Once actualized, it may then be recognized, addressed and worked through. It is persistent stasis that can indicate a problematic engagement and 'true' stuck point or 'bastion' in the process.

The illness of the Field

Stasis and repetition are not only inevitable, but they are desirable as way stations in the analytic process. The Field must, at some point, 'fall ill' if it is going to actualize and make present what needs to be worked through and resolved analytically. This is perhaps simply a re-statement in the language of a two-person psychology of Freud's (1914) comment regarding the transference that the enemy cannot be slain in effigy, or his description of how the infantile neurosis that produced the symptomatic neurosis is replaced by the transference neurosis and it is the latter that must be actualized if it is to be 'cured' in the analysis. (See also the many comments made by Winnicott (e.g. 1967, 1974) on the necessity to fail the patient in certain ways so that what was once suffered by an ego that could not yet hold together in the face of a traumatic rupture and failure of the facilitating environment, and so could not be 'experienced', could be brought into the here-and-now of the transference relationship and be 'experienced' for the first time.)

But if the Field is constructed by the unconscious of both parties, why is the cure directed towards only one of them? Certainly, it is possible that both participants will wind up better off for the experience of the analysis. To overemphasize this possible symmetry, however, would be misleading.

The analyst is bound by and the bearer of a psychoanalytic ethics: to be there in the service of the growth of the other and not the self (Chetrit-Vatine, 2004). It is not that analyst and analysand aren't 'symmetrical' in the sense of being humans in a relationship in which the rules of psychology must fall equally on the heads of all those present (Friedman, 1988). It is the analyst's subordination of self to the therapeutic/analytic needs of the other that creates an *ethically determined asymmetry* that tilts the therapeutic Field in the direction of the patient. And this is how it should be.

In addition, asymmetry preserves the enigmatic sense of the analyst as 'other-subject' (Roussillon, 2011), which remains a driving force in the analytic process. In this sense, the analyst's position is akin to a parent sacrificing for the developmental needs of their child, putting their own wishes and desires aside to some extent, but predominantly where the developmental needs of the child are concerned. This is not slavish submission or masochism. It is an act of sacrifice and love akin to that of the priestesses who served as the voice of the Oracle at Delphi. Once they entered the fire pit, they spoke in the service of the God. The words that emerged may have been spoken in a voice or dialect using metaphors drawn from a particular servant's personal experience, but the message that was conveyed was assumed to be not hers, but the God's. In the same way, the analyst's words and actions 'speak' *in the transference* (Sechaud, 2008) in the language of the patient's internal world. This 'speech' is always limited to some extent by the analyst's own subjectivity, but for the most part reflects the recruitment of the analyst into actualization of the conflicts of the patient.

A clinical illustration

First sequence

The patient, a single middle-aged man who suffers from isolation and schizoid withdrawal, has been in a four times per week analysis with a female analyst for many years. Towards the end of a session, which followed a cancellation initiated by the patient, he suddenly tells of an irritating event that occurred while waiting for a train. A young woman, whom he derisively refers to as 'narcissistic', ran over his foot with her luggage, didn't notice and just kept moving on without regard for the pain she had caused him.

Prior to his next session, he calls to say he will have to cancel. There had been a recent change in the session time initiated by the analyst, which the patient explains that his secretary at work didn't record and so the secretary booked something else in conflict with the new time that he now couldn't change. The analyst replies that the old time is actually still available that day, offers it to the patient and the patient agrees to come, but his agreement lacks enthusiasm. When this lack of enthusiasm is raised in the session, he agrees that yes, he is feeling indifferent about coming to analysis this day. He is depressed, hopeless, withdrawn, isolated, etc. He mentions his recently deceased father whom he feels has just 'disappeared' and his mother, who is slowly retreating further and further into dementia. The analyst comments that he seems to feel alone and without hope. He agrees.

A plausible Field hypothesis is that perhaps there has been an unexpected and untoward occurrence in the analysis, a jarring 'accident', that has gone unnoticed, leaving the patient feeling annoyed and neglected, much as one might feel when one's father dies and one's mother begins to disappear into dementia. The analyst's comment about the patient's feeling alone and without hope speaks directly to this dimension, without attempting to force narrative saturation or specific recognition or acknowledgment as a transference issue.

In the next session, a Monday, the patient continues by recounting how miserable and alone he was over the weekend. He expresses fears that he will lose his security clearance at work (i.e. bad things will be assumed or discovered about him) and that will lead to his losing his job. One thing he fears that might be misinterpreted is his need to be in analysis; another is the romance he had with a woman at his office in past years.

He imagines that he will be fired and complains that no one cares about or sees that he is doing a good job at work; that no one wants him. He becomes more depressed and hopeless. The analyst comments on this and attempts to make it more specific by adding, 'Perhaps you feel that here, too'. He says it is true of his mother, who gives him no warmth, but he doesn't think so here. At least here he can tell his analyst 'all of his shit' and get it off his chest. She is like the 'wailing-wall', where he goes to chant his misery.

He then begins to muse that something must be wrong with him, because everyone is always forgetting about him and neglecting him. He thinks of a hemiplegic friend, who desperately wants to move in with his girlfriend. The patient couldn't imagine feeling that way towards a woman, because he 'can't stand proximity'. But then he imagines a lonely, barren life in which he loses his job, walks his dog and drinks all day. 'Suicide lite' is what he calls it. His next thought is of the analytic relationship: 'How can you stand me for all these years? I say nothing new; it's the same things over and over again ...' Then he adds, 'You must be doing it for the money'.

One possible Field hypothesis is that perhaps the 'collision' referred to in the first session is related to the news of the change in appointment times. Or something the analyst said, did or did not sufficiently attend to or address earlier or in a previous session. The 'loss' of the second session and dispirited presentation may reflect the fact that the 'collision' wasn't recognized or commented on by the analyst (= the 'indifferent woman', who doesn't notice that she injured him; the disappearing and out of touch parents mirrored by the patient's own disappearance in failing to note the time change of the session).

We could also wonder if the analyst heard the story of fearing being rejected (losing his 'security' (!) clearance, fired) due to his anger at the 'narcissistic woman' (analyst) or his neediness and desire (*wanting* an affair; *needing* treatment) and the feeling that his good intentions (no one sees he is actually doing a good job) were not being noticed as a more saturated and organized signal about the transference. Hence her asking if the same wasn't going on in the analysis.

In addition, in perhaps unconsciously arranging to have to cancel his own session, is the patient retaliating or unconsciously asking the analyst to declare her interest by pursuing him, which she does by offering the still available old time? This 'countertransference action' from one perspective may therefore also be an actualization of the wished for pursuing and desiring object, as well as a concordant identification with the patient's own hungry pursuit of the analyst/parent. That is, an unconscious recruitment of the analyst into an enactment that turns up the volume of the signal of a particular constellation that is being actualized and brought forward in the Field.

In the Monday hour, the storm of hopelessness and neglect that the analyst had commented on gathers force, perhaps abetted by the weekend break. Characters, such as 'miserable and alone', 'loss of security', 'neediness' and 'desire' appear on stage, although their storylines have not yet begun to unfold with greater clarity or specificity.

In the third session, the patient again talks of being afraid of being 'found out' or seen in a particular way and fired [?by the analyst]. He would then wander and drink. Being alone feels like abandonment and leads to extreme defensive maneuvers of withdrawal and isolation that he calls 'suicide lite'. Yet, he also recognizes that unlike his friend who wants to have his girlfriend move in, he can't imagine or handle that much closeness. This leads to the appreciative recognition that the analyst has put up with his sterile repetition for many years, but the latter thought is quickly followed by pushing her away in the speculation that perhaps it is only his money that she is interested in.

The wailing-wall is an interesting 'character', not only for its reference to sadness, mourning and tears, but because it may be immovable (a wall), unless one has faith, in which case one can see it as a manifestation or location of God, a God who can answer one's prayers and the wishes (i.e. desires) of those who have need and faith and pray there. The patient doesn't say this, but in the analyst's associations, which are also a part of the Field, she recalls that in Jerusalem, people silently put written prayers into the cracks in the wall with the hope that they will be answered. Playing the Squiggle Game, the analyst might have commented to that effect. If so, what new movements and directions might that comment catalyze? Where might it lead to and whose 'construction' would it be? A comment about the Wailing Wall or the silent prayers that are placed there might take hold and function in the Field like Winnicott's (1971) reflex hammer, which he used to place in the visual field between himself and the infant he was examining. If the baby became interested in that object and began to explore it, visually or tactilely, then the hammer became the caesura that connected them and defined the location of the transitional space through which they were momentarily connected.

Second sequence

The patient, who had isolated himself and had been living a rather schizoid life, began a new romance and accepted an invitation from his girlfriend to come away on vacation. This will mean missing several sessions. He has just returned from a recent business trip to another country, where he was given a professional award. He begins by speaking about how different, how much better, the intellectual climate is in his profession in that other country; how much he enjoys learning and has benefitted from his travel.

His 'acceptance of learning' implies a part that is not entrenched in defensive omniscience and grandiosity. He can accept his ignorance and not knowing and without envying those who do know and therefore has a space to take in and learn [presumably in the analysis]. There is also the contrast between the limited home country [his self outside the session or prior to the analysis vs. the more intellectually competent 'new country' of his analysis?]. In other discussions, he has been keenly interested in what the analyst knows and does not know and was pleased when she recognized a literary reference he used in describing something.

His associations in the session move from the more stimulating, 'other country' to a book he is reading about Anthony Burgess, a man who came from a stimulating, rich English intellectual, upper class world, became a Russian spy and then defected to the (far more sterile) Soviet Union. He then thinks of his dementing mother, whose caretaker suggested that even without dementia had intellectual limitations. [The poverty of his 'home' country?]. He retreats from feeling by asserting he prefers to be alone and describes the pleasure of hanging lamps in his new house. [Having his own place rather than renting is new and quite pleasurable to him, and is also a step forward, as it is an investment in permanence and self; 'a room of his own'.]

He reasserts that he prefers to be alone and the analyst says: 'Maybe there is another feeling alongside that', implying that he also wants NOT to be alone; to be with someone.

His response is to report feeling restless and wanting to leave. He says he is looking forward to being alone on New Year's Eve as usual and prefers it this way. He next refers to his hanging the lamps as 'decorating a bomb shelter'. And how once on New Year's Eve, when he was renting, the landlord asked him to come to a party that he was giving and the patient refused.

In the back of the analyst's mind is the upcoming break for his beach vacation. She says: 'You want to withdraw, but you also regret the upcoming interruption. You didn't realize how many sessions you would miss here'. [That is, she hears his description of the party as relating to analysis and moves into a more saturated comment tying it more directly to the transference.]

He associates immediately to the title of the spy book, 'The LIVES of Burgess, plural'. And adds, 'Maybe I do have a second side. Now I regret that I'll be away for so long. I didn't realize how many sessions I will miss'. [Gambit accepted!]

The next session is complicated, in that it was on a Monday and at first the patient had once more canceled because of a work conflict. He then learned over the weekend that he could attend and sent a text to the analyst saying, 'I will be there Monday after all'. Her response was uncharacteristically brusque. She sent a text back saying 'Are you asking if it is still available?' He texted back, 'Yes please'. And she responded. 'It is OK as the time is still free.'

Just before he arrives for his session, the analyst realizes that she has forgotten to unlock the outer door. She hurries to do so minutes before he arrives! What is in the back of her mind when he arrives is that she has had a bad cold for several weeks and now the patient also has a cold. She assumes (consciously) that she wanted to lock him out to prevent him from blaming her for giving him the cold.

A new 'character' has appeared in the Field – located in the analyst – in the form of her unconsciously bristling at his expectation that the cancelled hour would still be available and 'forcing him' to acknowledge he wanted to see her by making the patient ask and not just assume he could come then. Then her annoyance becomes more forceful in her almost locking him out. Had he arrived and found the door locked, he would have had to express desire to enter by ringing or knowing and asking to be let in. The analyst's fantasy about being blamed, ostensibly for passing him her cold, is both a morality play – his – about the danger of contact with other humans and a presumed expression of her anger and a guilt reaction – hers – at her aggression, in forcing him to ask her and therefore show her his desire.

He opens the session by telling the analyst that he has been invited to a party by an ex-girlfriend. Can he get himself to attend? [Is the 'invitation' also to the analytic hour? Will he 'attend' and be more present and related in this session?] He associates to feeling happy and good in his new home. He's glad that he owns the house and is happy decorating it. But he describes an 'irrational fear' that the holes he has had to drill hanging the new lamps will weaken the structural supports of the house and cause a collapse. This is followed by a story of having been promised something by his old landlord, who then never followed through with payment. He has been reluctant to ask for what should rightly be his, for fear of being refused and an argument following. He summarizes it as follows: 'I don't want to be a beggar'. [Are these about the Monday hour and the dangers of 'attending' the session and being in greater emotional contact with the analyst and with himself? Is this the other side of the coin of the locked door and being forced to ask for the once cancelled appointment?]

His next associations are to how unacceptable and 'distasteful' he feels, with warts, fungus and a past history of an STD. He wishes his cold would quickly resolve, because he never wants to go to the doctor. When he was 12, his uncle accidentally slammed a car door on his hand and he still didn't want to go to the doctor. [Is this accident an emotional description of the negotiations over the return of the Monday hour? A more direct association to the earlier comment about being run over by the suitcase at the railway station? Is his ability to make or present unconscious symbolic links a reflection of his 'being in attendance?']

'That car door', he says, 'was my second castration'. (Earlier in life, there had been a surgery for phimosis). 'No, my third castration. When I was very young I had my ear-drum lanced because of an ear infection'. [No wonder he avoids and fears doctors! But aren't analysts doctors, too? 'Ouch!'] Then back to the novel of the spy who betrayed his country and betrayed himself. He was a lonely man who isolated himself because of his need to hide his homosexuality. [He does not say it, but the spy also wound up alone in Moscow, missing England terribly.]

Conclusion

While much of the brief clinical example that I have related can be understood from other contexts and perspectives, I have tried to show the potential value and some of the hypotheses that may be derived from attempting to read the discourse and interaction, from one man's subjective perspective, as presumptive signals from the Field. Of course, like any other hypotheses that emerge in the clinical situation, one must be circumspect and hold these to be presumptive and assumptive, ready to be evaluated for their utility and presumed meaning, re-evaluated and amended as subsequent developments occur. I believe that this 'GPS' dimension is the strength and value of the Field hypothesis, as long as it is tentative and remains open to emendation, correction and 're-routing'.

The final point I would like to make is that while I find the Field perspective to be of considerable value in my own clinical thinking, listening and work, I do not believe that its narratological co-constructive technical implications are always the only optimal response. As I use them, these remain in oscillating dialogue with other points of view that have become part of my analytic sensibility. In particular, I have found that the patient's capacity to use a co-construction of narrative approach must be predicated on the presence of a certain, unspecifiable degree of developed psychic capacity.

In other words, it takes someone who is willing and has the psychic capacity to play the verbal Squiggle Game with the analyst at any given time, if this interventional implication of the Field technique is to prove of value. While the GPS information of the Field is always potentially available to the analyst, the narrative co-constructive technique that can follow is not always the most useful. Patients who are deeply enmeshed in pathological organizations often need a preliminary period of explanation and confrontation before they can begin to develop or mobilize the psychic capacities needed to make use of narratological co-constructive interventions. That, however, is the subject of a separate communication.

Notes

1 An earlier version of this chapter appeared in Levine, H.B. (2016). A logica do campo [The logic of the Field]. *Revista de Psicanalise da Sociedade Psicanalitica de Porto Alegre*, 23: 255–280. We gratefully thank *Revista* for permission to revise and expand that publication.

2 My thanks to Jack Foehl and Chris Lovett, whose comments were of great help in the preparation of the final version of this manuscript and to the colleague who did the analysis and must remain anonymous for purposes of confidentiality.

3 Harry Stack Sullivan spoke of an interpersonal field (see Stern, 2013a, 2013b) and Robert Langs (1976) wrote of a bi-personal field, but while using the same word, 'field', these were significantly different concepts than the current one I am about to discuss and did not create a definitional consensus that established an agreed upon meaning for the term, Field. The question of their similarities to and differences from the current sense of Field Theory, derived from the work of the Barangers, Bion, Ferro and his colleagues, is beyond the scope of this paper.

4 In Spanish-language psychoanalysis, where the Field (*campo*) is a far more established and agreed upon concept, it has other antecedents in the work of authors such as Pichon-Riviere, who was influential in the thinking of the Barangers, but these are not part of the/my Anglophone context and so their contributions will reluctantly be left aside.

5 See Stern (2013a, 2013b).

6 The designations 'in' and 'of' the transference are commonly used in French psychoanalysis. For a description and discussion, see Sechaud (2008).

7 For an extended discussion of a revised epistemology for psychoanalysis, see Levine (2021).
8 See Freud's (1899) hypothesis that we may not have memories *from* childhood, only memories *about* childhood, and that the final form of these is determined by context and unconscious purpose and intent in the here-and-now.
9 See Rocha Barros and Rocha Barros (2011) for a detailed examination of symbols, symbol formation and symbolic forms.
10 See Kristeva (2001).
11 See also Levine (2015a).
12 Elsewhere, I have described this as a fundamental mental mechanism that I have called *The Representational Imperative* (Levine, 2013).
13 'Only the further course of the analysis enables us to decide whether our constructions are correct or unserviceable. We do not pretend that an individual construction is anything more than a conjecture which awaits examination, confirmation or rejection' (Freud, 1937, p. 265). See also Levine (2011).
14 For an anglophone description of this concept, see Scarfone (2015).
15 The inevitable repetition of successful working through is different in that the site of the repetition in the discourse may continually shift, as the same kind of conflict recurs inside, outside, in the present, in a dream or memory, etc.

References

Baranger, M. and Baranger, W. (2008). The analytic situation as a dynamic field. *International Journal of Psychoanalysis*, 89: 795–826.
Baranger, W. and Baranger, M. (2009). *The Work of Confluence: Listening and Interpreting in the Psychoanalytic Field*. Ed. by L. Glocer-Fiorini. London: Karnac/IPA.
Bion, W.R. (1961). *Experience in Groups*. London: Tavistock.
Bion, W.R. (1962). *Learning From Experience*. London: Heinemann.
Bion, W.R. (1963). *Elements of Psychoanalysis*. London: Heinemann.
Bion, W.R. (1965). *Transformations: From Learning to Growth*. London: Tavistock.
Bion, W.R. (1967). Notes on memory and desire. In *Melanie Klein Today*. Vol. 2: *Mainly Practice*. Ed. by E. Spillius. London: Routledge. pp. 17–21.
Bion, W.R. (1970). *Attention and Interpretation*. New York: Basic Books.
Bion, W.R. (1992). *Cogitations*. London: Karnac.
Bion, W.R. (2005). *The Tavistock Seminars*. London: Karnac.
Botella, C. and Botella, S. (2005). *The Work of Psychic Figurability: Mental States without Representation*. Hove and New York: Brunner-Routledge.
Chetrit-Vatine, V. (2004). Primal seduction, matricial space and asymmetry in the analytic encounter. *International Journal of Psychoanalysis*, 8: 841–856.
Edelman, G. (1989). *The Remembered Present: A Biological Theory of Consciousness*. New York: Basic Books.
Ferro, A. (2002). *In the Analyst's Consulting Room*. Hove and New York: Brunner-Routledge.
Ferro, A. (2005). *Seeds of Illness, Seeds of Recovery: The Genesis of Suffering and the Role of Psychoanalysis*. Trans. by Philip Slotkin. Hove and New York: Brunner-Routledge.
Ferro, A. (2006). *Psychoanalysis as Therapy and Storytelling*. Hove and New York: Routledge.
Freud, S. (1899). *Screen memories*. S.E. 3, pp. 299–322.

Freud, S. (1912). *Recommendations to physicians practising psycho-analysis.* S.E 12, pp. 109–120.

Freud, S. (1914). *Remembering, repeating and working through.* S.E. 12, pp. 145–156.

Freud, S. (1917a). *Introductory lectures on psycho-analysis III.* S.E. 16, pp. 243–463.

Freud, S. (1917b). *Mourning and melancholia.* S.E. 14, pp. 237–260.

Freud, S. (1923). *The Ego and the Id.* S.E. 19, pp. 109–124.

Freud, S. (1937). *Constructions in analysis.* S.E. 23, pp. 255–270.

Friedman, L. (1988). *The Anatomy of Psychotherapy.* Hillsdale, NJ: The Analytic Press.

Grotstein, J. (2009). Psychoanalysis as a passion play. In *The Analytic Field: A Clinical Concept.* Ed. by A. Ferro and R. Basile. London: Karnac. pp. 189–212.

Joseph, B. (1985). Transference: The total situation. *International Journal of Psychoanalysis,* 66: 447–454.

Kristeva, J. (2001). *Melanie Klein.* New York: Columbia University Press.

Langs, R. (1976). *The Bipersonal Field.* New York: Aronson.

Levine, H.B. (2010). 'The consolation which is drawn from truth': The analysis of a patient unable to suffer experience. In *Bion Today.* Ed. by C. Mawson. Abingdon: Routledge. pp. 188–211.

Levine, H.B. (2011). Construction then and now. In *On Freud's 'Constructions in Analysis'.* Ed. by S. Lewkowicz and T. Bokanowski with G. Pragier. London: Karnac. pp. 87–100.

Levine, H.B. (2013). The colourless canvas: Repetition, therapeutic action and the creation of mind. In *Unrepresented States and the Construction of Meaning.* Ed. by H.B. Levine, G. Reed and D. Scarfone. London: Karnac/IPA. pp. 42–71.

Levine, H.B. (2015a). Myth. In *The WR Bion Tradition.* Ed. by H.B. Levine and G. Civitarese. London: Karnac. pp. 307–314.

Levine, H.B. (2015b). Is the concept of O necessary for psychoanalysis? In *The WR Bion Tradition.* Ed. by H.B. Levine and G. Civitarese. London: Karnac. pp. 377–386.

Levine, H.B. (2021). *Affect, Representation and Language. Between The Silence and the Cry.* Abingdon and New York: Routledge.

Ogden, T. (1997). Reverie and metaphor. *International Journal of Psychoanalysis,* 78: 719–731.

Pirandello, L. (1998). *Six Characters in Search of an Author.* Trans. and Introduction by Eric Bentley. New York: Signet Classics.

Rocha Barros, E.M. and Rocha Barros, E.L. (2011). Reflections on the clinical implications of symbolism. *International Journal of Psychoanalysis,* 92: 879–901.

Roussillon, R. (2011). *Primitive Agonies and Symbolization.* London: Karnac/IPA.

Scarfone, D. (2006). A matter of time: Actual time and the production of the past. *Psychoanalytic Quarterly,* 75: 807–834.

Scarfone, D. (2015). *Laplanche.* New York: The Unconscious in Translation.

Sechaud, E. (2008). The handling of the transference in French psychoanalysis. *International Journal of Psychoanalysis,* 89: 1011–1028.

Stern, D.B. (2013a). Field Theory in psychoanalysis, Part I: Harry Stack Sullivan and Madeleine and Willy Baranger. *Psychoanalytic Dialogues,* 23: 487–501.

Stern, D.B. (2013b). Field Theory in psychoanalysis, Part 2: Bionian Field Theory and contemporary interpersonal/relational psychoanalysis. *Psychoanalytic Dialogues,* 23: 630–645.

Winnicott, D.W. (1967). The concept of clinical regression compared with that of defense organization. In *Psycho-Analytic Explorations*. Ed. by C. Winnicott, R. Shepherd and M. Davis. London: Karnac, pp. 193–199.

Winnicott, D.W. (1971). *Therapeutic Consultations in Child Psychiatry.* London: The Hogarth Press and the Institute of Psycho-Analysis.

Winnicott, D.W. (1974). Fear of breakdown. *International Review of Psychoanalysis*, 1: 103–107.

Chapter 3

Post-Bionian Field Theory

An illustration

Howard B. Levine

Bion (1962, 1970) elaborated a view of the psyche as potentially overwhelmed by internal and external stimuli, raw data, which must be psychically metabolized so that it can acquire subjective meaning and become the building blocks of thought. Failure to adequately do so leads to maladaptive, evacuative discharge phenomena, such as massive projective identification, hallucinosis, impulsive behavior, addictions, perversions, psychosomatic illnesses and other severe character pathologies. The origins of this raw data can be either internal (drives, as described by Freud) or external (sensory afferents, perceptions).

Central to the analytic process is Bion's contention that in addition to the patient's projective identifications serving a regulatory and defensive function for the individual and within the analytic couple or infant-caretaker dyad – a point that Melanie Klein had made early on – they also communicate distress, the need for assistance and *activate the psychic transformational capacities of the object*. (See also Aisenstein, 1993.) The analyst, in a state of reverie, one that tends towards non-tendentious listening aiming as much as possible to eschew memory, desire or specific theoretical expectations, absorbs the patient's projections and works upon (transforms) them unconsciously, so that they become capable of giving rise *in the mind of the analyst* to images, affects and ideas that will become the stuff of the analyst's thoughts, fantasies, etc. Having achieved psychic representation in the mind of the analyst, these images, affects and ideas may then be noticed and used by the analyst to either inform an interpretation or other comment that may or may not be given to the patient and/or to adjust the analyst's internal state, listening stance or perspective, degree of activity, etc.

The goals of analysis in post-Bionian Field Theory are transformational rather than informational. That is, rather than aiming predominantly at revealing what is hidden in the unconscious, analysis aims to create and expand the unconscious and the category of what is thinkable for the patient, starting with expanding what can be thought and felt within the analytic pair, and to strengthen and help develop the patient's capacity for tolerating and constructing their own thoughts and feelings. This applies to all phenomena, all 'capital E Experience',[1] across the full range of human possibility from the

DOI: 10.4324/9781003168034-3

autistic to the psychotic to the neurotic-normal. In this view, the work of analysis extends beyond the uncovering and 'decoding' of repressed, disguised and hidden meanings to include the intersubjective generation of affectively imbued thoughts that become organized into personal narratives and progressively linked to other thoughts, feelings and narratives.

Put in terms of technique, the interpretation of the here-and-now is not a 'destination', does not exhaust meanings, but is instead a point of departure for new meanings and places not yet known. 'Psychoanalysis is not a symbolic system charged with 'deciphering meaning', but a 'system for generating new thoughts' (Ferro and Basile, 2009, p. 92), which can then become progressively interlinked. This requires the creation and maintenance of a potential or unsaturated space, in which new thoughts may emerge. What this implies in terms of technique is that the analyst may use the fruits of his or her reverie and intuition to reply to the patient in the patient's idiom (within the terms and subject matter of the patient's manifest content), thereby participating in co-constructing a 'story line' as one might in play therapy with a child. With adults, however, instead of using toys or crayons and paper (as, for example, in Winnicott's Squiggle Game) to engage with, comment on and advance the patient's elaboration, the analyst uses words and the 'dialect' of the patient's manifest content.

Another central postulate in post-Bionian Field Theory is the assumption that in the analytic situation, the presence and activity of the analyst produces a continuing source of disturbance for the patient, which elicits the patient's ongoing response. This means that there is always a perspective from which the Field offers constant feedback about how the patient is unconsciously experiencing the analyst's presence, activity and the analytic situation. This perspective not only offers the analyst a continual source of data about the here-and-now of the analysis, but a continual opportunity to fine tune his or her response and activity as co-creator of the unfolding narrative texts of the session and co-regulator of the patient's emotional equilibrium within the session. It is important to note that the specific contents and meaning of this feedback are often enigmatic, obscure and subject to the interpretation of a given analyst and/or given analyst–patient pair. The interpretation and application of the lessons learned from the feedback is a subjective and intersubjective matter and therefore will be highly pair specific.

Post-Bionian Field Theory raises the technical question at every moment: 'What story can be told to and with the patient in order to help facilitate psychic growth and eventual understanding?' In traditional analytic formulations, the 'story' that analysts tell is called an interpretation and the related technical question has often been: 'Which interpretation of defense will allow the emergence of that which is split off, hidden or disguised?' Or 'Which interpretation of the unconscious will the patient be able to use or understand to reveal what is repressed or otherwise disguised?'

While these questions may be relevant for some patients at some moments, post-Bionian Field Theory offers other options as well. For example, before patients can use interpretations, they may first require assistance in elaborating upon and telling their story, so that there is a psychic content of significant symbolic value and meaning to interpret. In such instances, interventions aimed at facilitating the development of elements of thought or narrative sequences may be indicated before the analyst or patient is ready to step back and 'read' the implications of what has just been described.

It is also important to understand that in this theory, unlike in other psychoanalytic theories of technique, understanding and knowledge are not analytic ends in themselves. Rather, they are the means to the ends of catalytic transformation, psychic structuring and psychic change, the latter each being experiential process phenomena in the here-and-now. As Ferro (2006) described it:

> This, in my view, is the game of analysis: getting in touch with the entire unthinkable and unrepresentable world that was previously throbbing away amorphously, so as to confer on it a representation capable of 'narration', after which it will be capable of inhabiting an unconscious composed now of narratable, albeit repressed, elements of a story.
>
> (p. 108)

A brief vignette[2]

In the following material, I shall present a rather ordinary fragment of an hour of a patient's analysis, illustrating my assumption that patients' manifest discourse can be treated as their 'dream' of the session and the analytic relationship. I will emphasize my reading of the signals from the Field as they evolved within my mind during the hour and my attempts, conscious and unconscious, to use that reading to help the patient weave the fabric of a competent and expanding narrative. In particular, the material that I shall describe reflects my response to an unnoticed implication in the patient's discourse in which I unconsciously trigger and therefore introduce a covert reference to absence and loss that will reinforce an associative thread that runs through this patient's life and the material of the session.

Of course, other perspectives and formulations of the material are possible, as the material of the session may be assumed to be many other things: e.g. a true rendering of actual events in external reality; a disguised way of talking about the genetic past; a reflection of the patient's internal world; etc.

While the material selected may seem ordinary and perhaps even banal, it provides the basis for *my* 'dream' of the patient and indicates our work in the construction of *our* Field. What I hope to convey is a lively analytic process that we are unconsciously co-constructing, that is going on silently between and within each of us, and that I am consciously and internally tracking within the privacy of my own thoughts.

An academic in his early 50s, a child of survivors of the Holocaust whose beloved first wife died tragically of cancer many years before, begins an early morning analytic session on the couch, his second of three in the week, by praising the wonderful fall weather. [While this undoubtedly is an accurate description of something 'outside' of the analysis, it introduces an aura of pleasure, contentment in the Field and is presumably a comment on the current positive state of our relationship and the effects of the previous session.] His thoughts drift to the contrast between his happy new (third) marriage and his past conflicted (second) marriage from which he has only recently divorced. [According to the assumption that each character introduced in the patient's discourse also represents an affective presence within the Field, I hear this as referring to two possible pairings or 'weather systems': a benign 'marriage' (i.e. analytic relationship) and a malignant one. These may well represent potentially helpful and harmful moments building within the analysis, past, present and future.]

He next recalls that when he and his very problematic ex-wife, who was a writer, tried to work with their desks side by side, he was constantly distracted by their fighting or that the noise of her typing late at night disturbed his sleep. In contrast, his new wife can handle her business matters on her laptop without causing any disturbance. There are further references to various couples and pairs who were more successful in collaborating or in working together than he and his ex-wife.

[As he speaks, I am aware of how the rhythm of our work involves times when he seems to want and to do better on his own with less intervention from me – i.e. my metaphorical 'typing' (i.e. questions, observations and interpretations) disturbs his concentration – and other times, presumably now, when my activity is facilitating and/or less obstructive, and so we move more peacefully along in parallel. I assume that when seen from within the Field perspective, both pairs refer to us, but in the current moment, good pairing ('pleasant weather'; compatible third wife) seems to predominate.

This was my rather optimistic take on the moment, but in writing this, I would alternatively wonder if the analytic 'work' that my activity was fostering was the 'sleep disturbance' of his defensive denial and repression. Either? Both? Something else not yet recognized or formulated? Only patience and open-minded listening – Bion's 'negative capability' – will perhaps allow us to decide.]

As I continue to listen, I find myself associating to and beginning to feel personal thoughts and feelings of loneliness and loss. That is, a new 'weather front' has begun to gather in the Field, this time in the consciousness – or should we say *unconsciousness*! – of the analyst.

I privately reflect on the possible meanings of this new development and I wonder if my silent presence *at this moment in this hour* is enough to fulfill his 'side-by-side' wishes. That is, if his 'new wife'/analyst was not sufficiently felt to be present in the room, would he perhaps feel uneasy and miss her presence [weekend and other breaks in the rhythm of our meetings]?

I decide to shift my stance (I have been silent until now) and make a comment designed to both signal my presence, emotional as well as physical, and to test out and perhaps further elaborate my tentative formulation. However, like a play therapist in child analysis, I will keep my remarks within the idiom of his 'dialect' rather than asking about or calling direct attention to the 'meaning' or 'transference implications' of what he has just said. At the same time, in another part of my mind, I am silently aware of the possible transference connection I am about to make that, while I am not speaking in a way that will objectify and call attention to the transference, I am *speaking from within the transference.*[3] What I say is: 'So being close can be a mixed blessing. Sometimes it feels intrusive and disruptive, sometimes it just flows smoothly along'.

This comment seems to touch something, as he associates to the difficulties he has had as a single parent with two of his children [periods of time when there was no partner]. It is as if my saying 'being close' has activated feelings of its opposite, 'being alone', thereby introducing a new disruptive, irritating 'weather front' of 'absence', and has 'thickened' the plot. [He married his second wife in part in response to familial and internal pressure to give his children – and I think himself – a mother to replace his first wife who had died.]

He next speaks of his anger at his children's disruptiveness [perhaps an unconscious reference to my intervention and the distress caused by what it has reminded him of], his conflicts as a single parent – his first wife died of cancer when the children were still young – and he indirectly alludes to his guilt at times at having gotten so angry at his children [= perhaps the analyst, now?].

These comments lead to familiar descriptions of his parents' – especially his father's – pressure on him to remarry [perhaps he has heard my comment as a demand for him to move closer to/'marry' the analyst at *that* moment] for the children's sake after his first wife died, his resentment, his anger and his guilt. Guilt leads via association to the kind of man his Holocaust surviving father was: not like the all-American dads he saw on TV or the better integrated immigrant and survivor families that were cultured, educated and that he longed to belong to when he was growing up. [The two kinds of father are another reference to a contrasting closeness pair, like the contrast of the two wives earlier in the hour.]

As a further example, he refers to a local writer he met at a party, who had written an important book about the Holocaust and the second generation. My patient, who is an academic, has known about this book for some time and is surprised that he has avoided reading it. He asks: 'Do you think it would be good for me to read more about the Holocaust?'

[This question can be taken or heard at many levels. At the moment, I feel a closeness to him and assume that he has 'moved our desks side by side' and is addressing me in the father transference, to see if I will talk to him about what is unbearably painful. It is as if he has 'handed me the pen' and invited me to make a move in our Squiggle Game. I am the more Americanized father, the father he wished he had, the author he has 'met', the wife he can work alongside of, and he is considering risking letting himself be more open to my influence.]

Perhaps for some analysts, the 'orthodox' analytic response might be an inquiry into what he thinks or why he is asking me this at this time. These responses, each of them reasonable, lie within the context of a different theory. Intuiting/feeling/imagining that he has implicitly asked for help in expanding something inside of him, I simply say, 'Yes, although I am not saying that you *must* read them and I should also point out that given your interest in history and social science and how close this book is to your own experience, it may be noteworthy that you haven't read it so far'. (He has often read and talked about books that related to the immigrant experience, but not the Holocaust.)

His reply is an outpouring of description about how his mother, who had the rougher time of it during the war, almost never spoke about her war experiences, but then on rare occasions would show him a photo of her deceased sisters and brothers-in-law. I take this as his more specific introduction of a new set of characters – the ones who are never spoken of, the deceased, Auschwitz, where mother's relatives perished – and once more take up the metaphorical pen and add to our squiggle [i.e. introduce a more clearly emerging 'weather front' or set of characters into our discourse] by naming what has only so far been implied: 'The ones who were lost'. [This comment, through its non-specific reverberations, also links his first wife to the series.] 'Yes', he says and he recalls once more how his father would intermittently refer to his deceased family in a way that made my patient feel that they were a constant ghostly presence hovering in the wings of his family's life.

Now, these are facts of my patient's life that he has recounted many times before, without ever fully exploring and, in what I have silently assumed has been an identification with his child/self, I have *felt left out* of further understanding of the details of these events. I never felt that he felt that he could really do more than listen to his father – both parents are now deceased – and feeling my curiosity aroused, which I speculate may also be his, projectively received by me, I ask: 'When your father talked about them, was it the kind of talking that you felt allowed you to find out about father and his feelings and experiences? Or did you feel like it just pushed you away?'

[Although I am talking in the 'dialect' of the patient's manifest content, I am *at the same time and from a different perspective* also making a covert transference interpretation that takes into account the earlier signals about the two kinds of partnerships/marriages: the troubled relationship with the divorced ex-wife is linked in the patient's mind – or is it my mind? – with his troubled relationship with father and with the past and potential future troublesome moments in his relationship with me; the more successful working relationship links the more successful moments in the transference to his beloved deceased wife, the current wife and other positive and supportive figures, as symbolized by the kind of father who can invite you to talk with him about difficult, even horrible, things like the Holocaust and, since so much of our successful work has involved mourning the loss of his first wife, there is a link to her cancer and death, as well.]

Notes

1 See Chapter 2.
2 The patient's remarks will be described in the text. The analyst's reading of these remarks will be noted in square brackets.
3 The French make the distinction between interpretations *from within* the transference, in which the analyst's intervention is inevitably heard as if it was a line spoken in a transference drama, and interpretations *of* the transference, which name and objectify the transference by making a decoding statement, such as, 'you are reacting to me as if I was your father, when he ...' (see, for example, Sechaud, 2008).

References

Aisenstein, M. (1993). Psychosomatic solution or somatic outcome: The man from Burma. *International Journal of Psychoanalysis*, 74: 371–382.

Bion, W. (1962). *Learning From Experience*. London: Heinemann.

Bion, W. (1970). *Attention and Interpretation*. New York: Basic Books.

Ferro, A. (2006). *Psychoanalysis as Therapy and Storytelling*. Hove and New York: Routledge.

Ferro, A. and Basile, R. (2009). *The Analytic Field. A Clinical Concept*. London: Karnac.

Sechaud, E. (2008). The handling of the transference in French psychoanalysis. *International Journal of Psychoanalysis*, 89: 1011–1028.

Chapter 4

Dreaming upstream

Pictograms and the Field

Dolan Power

Bionian and post-Bionian Field Theory, richly creative and generative, provides us with a set of clinically useful concepts that mark out a particular territory amidst the wider array of intersubjective theories. Among what I consider to be the most useful of these concepts is that of the *pictogram*, a first transformation of raw beta (sensory) elements into pictorial or imagistic form and thus providing a crucial step in the movement from raw sensory experience toward thought and representation. When woven into narrations through the process of waking dream thought, these pictograms allow for thought, self-reflected experience (subjectivity), fantasy life, imaginal capacity, communicative projective identification and therefore intersubjective participation. As well, these processes of alphabetization and waking dream thought create a contact barrier that serves to distinguish and delimit conscious and unconscious mental life. In this chapter I explore the concept of pictogram, in hopes of extending and elaborating its theorization and applicability to certain clinical problems, the sources of which lay 'upstream' (Civitarese and Ferro, 2013; Ferro, 2009a, 2009b, 2012, 2015) and therefore closer to the body and early sensory experience. Problems originating in these areas are more likely to arrive in the consulting room in ways that are variously clamorous, silent, chaotic, unintegrated, fragmented and/or in action. In Ferro's view, deficits arising in this vaguely designated area call for extra measures by the analyst, and place extra psychic burdens upon her, in the service of stimulating and promoting the more usual downstream operations where communicative projective identification, waking dream thought, co-narrative exchange, and dreams-for-two (Cassorla, 2013) signal the presence of the patient's more robust alpha functioning. Referring to the challenges facing the analyst working in areas of the psyche where these capacities are less well established, Ferro (2009a) states that when the proto-emotional states are unalphabetized and fragmented, for example when the patient is silent,

> the analyst must himself perform *operations upstream* of the container/ contained, Ps-D and NC-SF, and form a-elements from agglomerations of B-elements. The analyst can get in touch with these a-elements either

DOI: 10.4324/9781003168034-4

by means of his reverie or progressively through dialogue and exchange of emotions (even small quanta of B – a) constructed in the relationship with the patient.

(pp. 85–86, italics added)

Through an extended clinical example I argue for broadening the concept of pictogram to include psychic processes thought to occur at the very earliest moments of psychic life and hypothesized to color the earliest renderings of somatic life into proto-mental experience, a subjective coloration that lends (or fails to lend) psychic life a vitality and investment in furthering its own continued growth and development. I argue that failures at this earliest of stages in the development of pictograms may be one source of difficulties, subsequently observed in the Field, of downstream operations.

In essence I argue for including in our understanding of the concept of pictogram the one offered by Piera Aulagnier (1975), who felt that the integration of sensory life was the basis and beginning of early psychic life, and who emphasized the importance of 'irradiating pleasure and auto-engenderment', and vicissitudes in these processes. Though not a Field theorist. and while coming from an entirely different psychoanalytic tradition, her contributions allow for an extension and elaboration of the pictogram concept in ways highly useful for understanding and working with those difficulties Ferro nominates as sourced 'upstream'. My goal in this chapter is to inform and enrich our understanding of the concept of pictogram as we might use it in the contemporary psychoanalytic Field.

Ferro's pictogram

While acknowledging Aulagnier's earlier use of the term 'pictogram', da Rocha Barros (2000) introduces a new definition for the term pictogram. In his re-definition, he draws on Ferro's (1995, p. 133) use of the phrase *dream-like photogram of the waking state*, which he uses to refer to an affective hologram of the analytic couple described as a syncretic designation of emotions. Drawing on the definition of *pictogram* in Paul Robert's dictionary (1984) that refers to the translation of ideas into figurative and symbolic scenes, da Rocha Barros, shifting the emphasis away from the *translation of ideas* and toward the *transformation of emotions*, states:

I use pictogram in a related way, to refer to a very early form of mental representation of emotional experiences, fruit of the alpha function, which creates symbols by means of figurations for dream thought, as the foundation for, and first step towards, thought processes. Strictly speaking, however, pictograms are not yet thought processes, since they are expressed in images rather than in verbal discourse and contain powerful expressive-evocative elements, but are very different from beta elements

(Bion, 1963)which are raw elements due to be expelled from the mental apparatus, when they are not transformed by the alpha function into alpha elements.

(De Rocha Barros, 2000, p. 1094)

This definition of pictogram seems to have been adopted by Ferro as reflected in his 2002 article discussing implications of Bion's thought. Ferro writes:

My point is that the patient 'responds' to every emotional movement of the analyst by producing a pictogram in real time, and the 'response' is also a narrative derivative of the waking dream thought – that is, of the sequence of alpha elements pictographed in response to the interpretive stimulus.

(p. 601)

This is a pictogram that is produced in real time during the immediate experience of the analytic process. It is the end product of gathering beta elements and metabolizing them into a representational image. They are visual and imagistic images of alphabetized beta elements which form a necessary foundation for the dreaming ensemble (Grotstein, 2009, p. 746). Ferro and Civitarese (2015) state: 'We all have an 'inner painter' who transforms primitive sensoriality into images and pictograms ... equating analysis with the aesthetic experience, it is possible to help the patient reach a fuller sense of consonance and contact between mind and body' (Ferro and Civitarese, 2015, p. xvii). They elaborate by connecting the term pictogram to Bion's description of how the mind functions in response to sensory input: 'Bion provided us with a model of the mind involving a continuous production of images (that could be called pictograms) by a function (described as alpha function) on the basis of the sensoriality that pervades us from whatever source' (p. 14).

Over time this use of the definition of the term pictogram has variously come to also include the phrases 'affective pictograms' or 'emotional pictograms'.

Aulagnier's pictogram

Aulagnier's book *The Violence of Interpretation* (1975) was an important intellectual statement and a public announcement of her separation from Lacanian psychoanalysis. Andre Green had already published an article on negative capability in 1973, and was generating interest in more primitive mental experience. Aulagnier's work married a growing French interest in an unconscious embedded in the body with an articulation of the infant's developing subjectivity and capacity for representational activity, using this understanding to inform analytic work with psychotic patients. Put another way, while Winnicott gave us a Google map of the mother–infant couple and what the real presence of the object means for the baby's development,

Aulagnier's theory of the pictogram gives us access to a zoomed-in view of the richness and aliveness of what may be happening psychically during that iconic Winnicottian period when 'there is no such thing as a baby'. In *The Violence of Interpretation*, Aulagnier describes the infant's psychic development during this period we characterize with phrases like, going-on-being, holding, normal maternal madness and harmonious interpenetrating mix-up, to name a few. Central to Aulagnier's (1975) theory of this earliest period of development is her concept of the **pictogram**:

> If I have chosen the initial experience of an experience of pleasure as the starting point of my construction it is because of the function that I give sensory activity, the original source of *pleasure* (of taste, hearing, seeing, feeling, touching) *which is the condition and cause* of the cathexis of a physical activity that the psyche discovers in its power – an experience of a pleasure that it obtains, which is *the necessary prerequisite for the cathexis of the activity of representation and of the image that results from it.*
>
> (p. 24, emphasis in the original)

Aulagnier is implying here that investment is not just investment in using the senses and not just the experience of bringing about pleasure, but she is stressing an investment in the pleasure of sensing. Or to put it another way, it is not only that one is excited by what one sees or tastes but that one is excited by the act of seeing, the function of seeing or tasting. In this way, pleasure is a function and the result of a function, a capacity and the result of a capacity. She is highlighting the discovery of a power 'to see, to hear, to feel, to touch, to taste', which will be metabolized by the psyche in the representation of its power to produce for itself the object and the state of pleasure. She refers to the process of 'self-engenderment' in describing a self to self-sensory experience. This is different from the idea that the infant is internalizing a capacity from the object. The object's role is to be a background presence that supports but does not impinge. Aulagnier introduces the term 'pictogram' to refer to the representation of this 'sensory-object-zone as the cause of excitation' by an image that presents them as a single, inextricable entity. It is this entity that she calls 'the image of the corporal thing'. **This image is the pictogram**. And its development, reflective of a beginning capacity for what, by its nature, is felt to be self-initiated representation (tinged with qualities that are pleasurable or unpleasurable), is an important marker on the way towards the subjectivation of experience.

Aulagnier's writing is dense and difficult to understand but she is basically describing that at the beginning of psychosomatic life (the primal), the pictogram is the earliest effort *toward* representation and that it is a function of bodily experience, rather than experience with an object perceived as such.

In the bodily experience of the mouth/breast or zone/object encounter the pictogram is formed by the infant psyche presenting experience to itself as if created by itself (what Aulagnier calls *self-engenderment*) during the phase of development that precedes object relating. The role of the object is more in keeping with Winnicott's (1958, p. 33) environmental mother or Grotstein's (2009, p. 14) background object of primary identification. Aulagnier tells us that at birth the psyche registers information from the body and derives life-enhancing pleasure from doing so. All the while the mother is safeguarding this earliest experience of agency by providing an 'irradiating pleasure' that bathes the baby in a pleasurable feeling which enhances the baby's feeling of self-agency. This leads to what she refers to as an early pictogram of either 'conjunction' or 'rejection'.

Joyce McDougall in her preface to Aulagnier's (1975) *The Violence of Interpretation* describes the two types of pictograms in the following way. When the encounter is associated with pleasure, the representation, in Aulagnier's terminology, is the 'pictogram of conjunction', representing the conjunction of the erogenous zone and its complementary object (based on the prototype of the mouth–breast conjunction), the whole being experienced as self-engendered and self-devouring. When feelings of displeasure or pain do not permit this pictogram, the experience is then treated with total rejection: rejection of the erogenous zone and its complementary part object, as well as the psychic activity which believes it has engendered the experience. Thus not only is the subject totally excluded from the psyche, but so is the representation and the experience itself. This creates what Aulagnier names the 'pictogram of rejection' (ibid., p. xx).

This early pictogram of either 'conjunction' or 'rejection' is a foundational experience of registering sufficient bodily pleasure or its deficit; unpleasure. Aulagnier is stressing the earliest experiences of the baby's relationship to its bodily self, and in this way her thinking is closer to the Winnicottian (1966) notion of psyche-soma indwelling, or Ferrari's (2004) vertical axis and the elaboration of Ferrari by Lombardi (2002, 2008). For all of these authors there is a basic agreement with Aulagnier that 'the body is the hero, the author of the psyche' (Flanders, 2015, p. 1406).

Aulagnier's pictograms of conjunction and rejection

For Aulagnier the infant must experience the 'irradiating power of pleasure' which lights up the nascent bodily self with an interest in investment or the taking in of pleasure/life. This investment in taking in life indicates that a pictogram of conjunction is dominant and results from a more or less seamless maternal provision of what is necessary/needed by the baby.

Here the pictogram of conjunction is embedded in the bodily-self experience of pleasure. The complementary object-zone (mouth–breast encounter) is experienced by the infant as pleasure given to the self by the self. The object and self are inextricably one. In fact, the phrase 'object and self' has no meaning at this level. The infusion of pleasure from the mother stimulates the baby's sensory activity (of taste, hearing, seeing, feeling, touching) and thereby ignites the self's investment in investing in using the senses. Specifically, this is not just an investment in sensorial pleasure, but rather, a pleasure and investment in the pleasure of sensing. Aulagnier elaborates: 'The discovery of a power "to see, to hear, to feel, to touch, to taste", which will be metabolized by the psyche in the representation of its power to produce for itself the object and the state of pleasure' (1975, p. 25).

This is different from the idea that the infant is internalizing a capacity from the object. According to Aulagnier the object's role is to be a background presence that supports but does not impinge upon the infant's experience of self to self pleasure, and thereby enables a sense of agency to take root within the infant. During this earliest period of life, which Aulagnier refers to as 'the primal', feeling is synonymous with experiencing the self. Therefore to experience pleasure is equivalent to feeling oneself as pleasurable. This bodily feeling is the bodily representation of what will in the later developmental phases of the 'primary' and 'secondary' be represented in words and then via symbolic fantasy.

When there is not enough infusion of necessary pleasure the baby is bathed in displeasure and suffering resulting in a 'pictogram of rejection'. Too much or too long experience of unrelieved states of suffering have disastrous effects on the process of investment in investing or taking in from outside the self. The ensuing bad feeling is experienced as a bad self and results in a mode of keeping out rather than taking in and can become fertile ground for the development of entrenched self-hatred.

This not taking in results in withdrawal from the world and most importantly leads to a sensory process of disinvestment leaving the infant with a preponderance of unmetabolized and unrepresented primordial experience of displeasure which has the potential to burden ensuing self and other experience. I will come back to this later in discussing the clinical example. Aulagnier's pictogram offers early, upstream understanding of the trouble dreaming in Ferro's Field. The body brings unmetabolized/unrepresented experience into the Field via bodily actions and bodily complaints derived from the first Field of experience of the earliest baby/mother experience which has been dominated by pain and displeasure. In this way the early pictogram of rejection is brought to the analyst for repair and acceptance.

Melissa: Clinical material

The early months of analysis with Melissa were especially difficult. Although she had attended a prestigious university and demonstrated considerable artistic talent, Melissa had spent her post-college years withdrawn in her room while living with her parents. Often she found it impossible to leave the house. The family rarely saw her as she usually isolated herself in her room with the door shut. Her mother finally sought another round of help for Melissa when she was in her mid-20s. There had been previous failed thera- pies dating back to childhood. Usually therapy ended because the therapist felt they could not be of help to Melissa. I began seeing Melissa five times a week face-to-face and I learned from her that she had never felt like she fit in at home or at school. She complained of noises in her head, noises she experienced sometimes as searing pain. She felt her last therapist had been nice but didn't know how to help her. Melissa had been diagnosed with ADHD as a young child and she remembers school as a place where teachers yelled at her to get control of herself and nobody liked her. Her parents cur- rently felt she wasn't trying hard enough to advertise her considerable artistic talents or to develop a social life. She had tried a psychiatric day program for anxiety but eventually lost interest in keeping up with the behavioral techni- ques. She felt easily assaulted by noises, visual stimulation, or people around her. During our first meeting she told me:

> Life feels very loud … just very loud … loud everything. Or it's … it's like … I mean it's wrong … the way the outside world is wrong. Even if it's not people … it's wasteful, clumsy and it ends up being harmful. I know I'm not apart from that … I'm gross. Just feel it overwhelming … don't know how to … I can't even keep a hold of my own life. I don't know where to start when there … is anything else around me.

She didn't like to drive and arrived late for her second appointment in a storm of frustration and rage. She screamed in frustration to the point that I felt embarrassed and had a powerful urge to tell her to 'get control of herself' so that colleagues in my suite wouldn't hear her. Perhaps this was my begin- ning identification with her and with her objects. Was I beginning to take in some important aspect of her experience – of deep shame and exposure? I wondered about a defensive wish projected into 'my colleagues' that I did not want to 'hear' (meaning take in), her wild and furious thoughts and feelings. She was beside herself that she was late and hadn't been able to find a parking place. In addition to this, she managed to convey to me, in fits or bursts of halting words, that all of this meant she was once again failing at therapy. She couldn't do anything right so what was the point? This feeling of failing, futility and frustration has remained a constant backdrop in the analysis. A backdrop that can recede temporarily but is inevitably evoked and experi- enced, usually in response to a felt demand to speak or think. During this early period of the analysis I learned that she was hitting herself and screaming at home. Her bruised legs and arms were evident in sessions. Her parents wondered whether analysis was making her worse and complained that she wasn't working and wasn't trying hard enough to make friends, but instead always pushed people away. There was a constant threat that her parents would stop treatment. Melissa herself became increasingly non-verbal in sessions, often falling asleep and when awake seemed to struggle to speak. When she did find words it was to shout at me that 'nothing was helping, this isn't helping!' Sometimes she would hit her shoulders and legs with her fists. At other times Melissa was able to talk for brief periods. She let me know that although she knew her parents were frightened by her hitting and screaming, in the moment she had no warning and that this behavior was unpredictable. This left her feeling that she never knew who she was minute to minute. This was one of the reasons she didn't like to be around other people. She had been hitting herself in private for many years. I was filled with great concern for her and constant anxiety that the analysis would be stopped before it had a chance to start. There were times that Melissa was remarkably articulate and expressive. For example, once during a joint meeting with her parents, she said to her mother, 'Why did you let me slip away?' Although her mother responded by acknowledging that she hadn't been as attuned as she should have been, there was a painful lack of feeling in her words. Melissa described her mother as someone who 'wasn't so good with just hanging out' or 'she's not so compassionate'. I heard Melissa unconsciously telling me that slipping away from the object was an ever-present danger and that in our work together her confidence in a secure and loving connection would be a fragile connection. Given my own constant concerns about the fragility of the treatment, our mutual immersion in the intersubjective Field forced on us disturbing feelings of discontinuity, ongoing unpredictability and searing pain. From Aulagnier's perspective we can imagine Melissa as someone who experienced too much suffering or unpleasure during the primal and that her autistic defenses (withdrawal into a bodily, sensory immersion), and historical preference for being alone are present day footprints of her pictogram of rejection. My reveries were sparse or nonexistent. I primarily felt an ongoing sense, heightened when Melissa was either sleepy, or awake but frustrated and unable to find words, that each session was the last session and that she wouldn't return. I was finally able to step back from this experience and begin to wonder whether Melissa might be communicating to me her fear, really more like her conviction, that I wouldn't return for the next session and couldn't tolerate her desperate need for help and that my words didn't help. I felt intense feelings of rejection and that I was a bad analyst. There seemed to be no way to gain entrance into Melissa's world in any sustained way. Often, I felt I was beginning to make contact with her in a session only to feel like a door was slammed in my face during the next session. One day Melissa arrived and said in an unusually organized and direct way that she was worried that she had parked her car in a spot where she might be towed due to street cleaning. She asked me if the street cleaners had already come by. I said I wasn't sure and that their schedule was not always predictable. I was heartened that Melissa was communicating her anxieties in words and making a direct request for my help. I asked her if she'd like to go back to her car and make sure she was in a safe spot. Surprisingly, she vigorously shook her head no. It seemed silly to go ahead with the session in a way that might ask Melissa to put aside a real anxiety about her car being towed. When she shook her head 'no' I could see real fear in her face. Responding to her fear I asked if she'd like to go together and she immediately agreed. We got up and walked around the corner from my office. I saw a couple of construction workers and asked if the street cleaners had been by and promptly learned that they had. Melissa was visibly calmed by this news and we quickly returned to my office. Once she sat down in her chair, she looked at me directly and murmured softly, 'Thank you for helping me'. Why was Melissa grateful and what had actually helped analytically beyond clarifying the real situation of whether her car was in danger of being towed? I think of this episode as indicating that Melissa was operating on a fairly concrete level of action in communicating her request for help. And at the time I heard it as a concrete request that I felt important to acknowledge and respond to because it was being expressed in words (which was highly unusual) and because this was the first time she was making a request for help directly to me. Later, after the session and in the weeks following the incident, I came to understand it, also, as Melissa's plea for my help in securing a place for her bodily self with me, in the analysis. Thought of this way, her request conveyed a profound anxiety about losing herself or being annihilated (i.e. the street cleaners coming) if she parked herself in the analytic space of my office. She was communicating an experience of being untethered in her own bodily/ parking place and worried about being lost (towed) because there would be no object to hold on to that would also hold onto her.

Aulagnier's ideas regarding the importance of the mother's irradiating pleasure bathing the baby in a pleasurable bodily experience that is felt to be self-engendered [the area of the primal] seemed to me to more accurately describe the level from which Melissa's difficulties arose. I began to wonder whether Melissa was bathed in profound displeasure which led to an experience of auto-engendered self-hatred and a profound feeling of rejection. From the perspective of Field Theory, Melissa's deficits – here I am referring specifically to the frailty of her capacities to communicate her experience verbally, her self-abuse, her frank withdrawal through silence, drowsiness and all manner of actual interpersonal/ social withdrawal, her apparent lack of fantasy and dream life and the marked constriction of my reverie life during sessions – suggest (in Field Theory terms) that her difficulties are located 'upstream'. Stated otherwise, the difficulties with which she struggles have their origins at a level which disrupts a basic capacity to 'author' one's initial sensory experience and integration in such a way that it is colored in a pleasurable, positive and life-enhancing palette (I take as a given that this process always assumes the presence of a maternal surround). Downstream, the disturbance is reflected in difficulties in mutual, intersubjective processes between patient and analyst, and the burden for making meaning of raw experience (transformations of experience via the oneiric dream spectrum) fall disproportionately and severely on the analyst. In these clinical situations communications from patient to analyst are heavily burdened by evacuative demands rather than communicative ones. This results in a deficit in dreaming.

Melissa and I were not yet at a level Cassorla (2013) refers to as 'dreams-for-two' but working at a level better characterized as 'doing-for-two', which involved a hybrid state of some ability to verbalize a need for help to sort out a confusing reality (whether her car was safe from towing) and some ability to welcome the presence of another (we went together) in joint action addressing the need for help. I think this is as an example of when the analytic challenge is to 'dream' privately, while responding in a concrete way to the patient, but followed by the analyst's continued dreaming the patient into existence outside of the session which is then brought back to the analytic work. I now understand this as a working together that could be thought of as more 'successive approximations' than of 'guided precision'. The parking space exchange illustrates this process, one that I think of as unfolding, spiraling and organized by a kind of GPS-like signaling that is not so much under the aegis of a symbolized communicative exchange but more so an exchange of simple concrete actions. I think of Melissa telling me she doesn't feel she has 'parked her car in a safe spot' and my suggestion that *she go herself and check on it* as missing the level of anxiety she was experiencing. When I offer to accompany her she can feel her place with me to be more secure. I am hearing her request not just at an object relational level, but at a deeper level, which I associate with Auglanier's level of the primal and the pictogram of rejection. In this way I'm beginning to *dream* (give meaning to) her experience as one in which she doesn't have *a place within herself* that is secure (sturdily integrated, anchored and hence safe) because of the pictogram of rejection – and so it is constantly threatening to be the dominant experience of the analytic encounter – an experience more atmospheric/spatial than object related. In this way of thinking the office instantly 'became' the bodily experience of Melissa (at the primal level, there is no 'Otherness', meaning that the object and physical surround and the sensory/somatic/psychic are identical, equivalent and auto-engendered). The forcefulness characteristic of her complaints and distress now seemed less like communications and more akin to evacuations, that is, closer to bodily expressions of somato-psychic irritation and distress.[1] I think that at the level of the primal the responsibility of the analyst is to hear the concreteness of the patient's experience while maintaining a private capacity to 'dream' that is held very conservatively so as to not force the patient to deal with a higher level of functioning that would only replicate the early mother–infant traumatic impingement. In time Melissa began to work, registered for an evening college course, and began to paint and decorate her room at home. She explained to me that her mother had painted her room a color she hates when she moved out for college. She loves the new color on her walls. I am analytically heartened by these changes and hear them (dream them) as a sign the analysis is helping despite the extremely difficult process in the analysis. This indicated to me that there was positive movement in Melissa's self-engenderment of a more positive pictogram, one of conjunction rather than rejection. She is experiencing her room/body space as a space that is filled with pleasure, i.e. she likes the color. This pleasure, this aesthetic appreciation, has very deep somato-sensory roots, constantly and repeatedly self-engendering a positive experience of the self. One could hear this material at a higher, more object relational level of Melissa asserting autonomy and feeling entitled to choose the color of her own walls rather than submit to her mother's preference. One could also hear it as a reference to the transference, as if she were saying to me, 'your office is so comfortable and I feel good being here with you because I increasingly feel that I have a say'. While these readings may capture some important aspects of Melissa's experience, I think that at this point in Melissa's treatment these 'meanings' are best kept to the margins of our clinical thinking and approach. To do otherwise, to move them more to center stage clinically (and I believe this is always our tendency) would be to misunderstand Melissa's level of symbolic functioning and capacity to experience the 'as if' quality of the transference. I think this kind of misunderstanding may be one of the reasons previous therapists felt they could no longer help her. There was a tendency to interpret her actions and expect her to relate at too high an object relational level when she is operating predominantly in the area Winnicott refers to as 'indwelling of the psyche in the soma' or Aulagnier's primal. As I thought back to the episode regarding her parked car and her fear that it would be towed, I was heartened to begin to understand a coherency in being with Melissa. Despite the ever present background of misery, bad feeling, confusion, and loss I could now see that Melissa was doing the best she could to communicate where and how she felt she had a place/self and her deep anxieties about not having a self or losing her place/self. There had been overall a nebulous movement in a more positive and articulated direction that might be viewed as strengthening her upstream operations in the hopes of being able to generate dreaming in the Field down the line. But as of yet, dreaming has not been possible, until there is a foundation strengthened in the body/self as anchored to perceptual experience, Melissa is vulnerable to 'losing' herself through dissociation, or a false self-presentation when in the presence of others.[2]

A short while later Melissa arrived for her session dressed in flowing long pants and a floral jacket with make-up, hair washed, combed and done in contemporary fashion. During this session she spoke about how she loved sewing her own clothes or looking for one-of-a-kind pieces in used clothing shops. Dressing in ways she liked was a way she brought joy to herself. It made her feel good and she thought it was a way of communicating something about her self to the world. In a subsequent session she spontaneously brought up that she was considering a promotion to a supervisor position at her place of employment. She explained that she would make only a little bit more money but that it would look good on her resume if she wanted to look for a different job in the future. She thought she was pretty good at dealing with frustrating people and better than her boss who just growled at people. She described how she was feeling more confident in herself. The new position meant working more hours and dealing with more frustrating people but maybe that might be a good thing. I commented that it sounded like she was surprised at her own capacity and that the job had brought out strengths she didn't know she had. She thought this was true.

Discussion

I have tried to elucidate the need to augment Bionian and post-Bionian Field Theory's use of the pictogram with the conceptualizations of Piera Aulagnier's pictogram. The integration of these two uses of pictogram would broaden the clinical sensitivity of the analyst working with patients whose problems lie 'upstream' and who are not yet capable of dreaming with the analyst on the level that Ferro describes as reflecting greater 'downstream' capacities.

At the level of sensory/somatic integration, the primal level, the communication is more about a gap in the ongoing sense of auto-engendered unity of pleasurable experience, a gap that engenders instead an experience of disharmony and unpleasure. In this way, Aulagnier's pictogram of rejection can bolster analytic understanding of those patients whose difficulties originate in the earliest phase of development of psychic life. Often these patients are action prone, without words sufficient to express and contain their experience, difficult to connect to and prone to respond with refusal to the analyst's attempt to generate an analytic process via dreaming-for-two. We can now understand that the trouble 'upstream' that prohibits dreaming, that they are now bringing to the analyst for repair, is a pictogram of rejection via unmetabolized/unrepresented bodily experience of pain and displeasure derived from traumatic early infantile experience. For example, this is how I now view Melissa's initial screaming and bouts of hitting herself. This 'proto-emotional storm' indicated that she had developed little alpha function to bring to bear on her deep frustration and pain. Her constant lament that 'words don't work' or 'I can't do this' can now be viewed as her best effort to convey to me the disruption in her earliest infantile experience. Was she saying, 'words don't work with me because they impinge on my experiencing pleasure as a pleasure given to myself by myself'? Likewise her lament early on to me that her mother lacked 'compassion' and 'wasn't so good at just hanging out' were present-day echoes of an early pictogram of rejection rather than a pictogram of conjunction. Is Melissa telling me about her lack of an environmental mother whose job is to provide a surround of good enough satisfaction, but most importantly, a feeling of loving pleasure that enables the infant to experience seamlessly a pleasure that is experienced as self-engendered? It is through this developmental process that a sense of agency is built; the baby needs to first feel seamlessly supported by an environmental mother who infuses the baby with pleasure that the baby experiences as actively given to the self by the self. This is a vital and necessary experience of pleasure infused by the environmental as the self giving pleasure to the self. This is Aulagnier's pictogram of conjunction. Melissa's early request that I go with her to check that her parking spot was safe is in action and outside of the consulting room. Aulagnier's use of the pictogram now gives a useful way to analytically conceptualize what felt intuitively right to me in the moment. I offered Melissa help to go together. This was not a dream-for-two, but rather a doing-for-two on behalf of one. By this I mean I now understand Melissa as thanking me for helping her to feel more anchored in herself and secure in her body/place. I am not hearing her expressed gratitude as thanking me for giving help contributing to a relationship between us. This experience was more one of appreciating my actively modifying the conditions of our contact, contact that carried the hazards of catastrophic loss and annihilation of the self arising from the impingement of an Other not attuned to the level of her anxieties when faced with the presence of the object. One cannot overestimate the natural analytic inclination to experience these kinds of patients' communications as organized on a more mature object relational level and connoting greater symbolized interpersonal meaning than in fact they are. The countertransferential pitfalls related to working with this level of pathology are many. Broadening our theoretical and conceptual understanding and our clinical use of the pictogram to include Aulagnier's ideas can be of great help to the analyst in deconcretizing the very chaotic, bodily, action-prone forms of communication and provide creative containment for these 'upstream' areas appearing in the analytic process.

Notes

1 For a discussion of evacuative projective identification as a communicative signal, see Bergstein (2015).
2 Though working from different psychoanalytic traditions, Winnicott's and Auglanier's concepts share a considerable affinity and overlap with each other.

References

Aulagnier, P. (1975). *The Violence of Interpretation: From Pictogram to Statement.* London: Routledge.

Bergstein, A. (2015). Attacks on linking or a drive to communicate? Tolerating the paradox. *Psychoanalytic Quarterly*, 84 (4): 921–942.

Bion, W. (1963). Elements of psycho-analysis. In *Seven Servants.* New York: Aronson. pp. 22–27.

Cassorla, R.M. (2013). When the analyst becomes stupid: An attempt to understand enactment using Bion's theory of thinking. *Psychoanalytic Quarterly*, 82 (3): 323–368.

Civitarese, G. and Ferro, A. (2013). The meaning and use of metaphor in analytic Field Theory. *Psychoanalytic Inquiry*, 33 (3): 190–209.

da Rocha Barros, E.M. (2000). Reflections on the clinical implications of symbolism. *International Journal of Psychoanalysis*, 81 (6): 1087–1099.

Ferrari, A.B. (2004). *From the Eclipse of the Body to the Dawn of Thought*. London: Free Association Books.

Ferro, A. (1995). *A Tecnica na Psicanalise Infantil*. Rio de Janeiro: Imago.

Ferro, A. (2002). Some implications of Bion's thought: The waking dream and narrative derivatives. *International Journal of Psychoanalysis*, 83 (3): 597–607.

Ferro, A. (2009a). *Mind Works: Technique and Creativity in Psychoanalysis*. New York and Abingdon: Routledge.

Ferro, A. (2009b). Transformations in dreaming and characters in the Field. *International Journal of Psychoanalysis*, 90 (2): 209–230.

Ferro, A. (2012). Creativity in the consulting room: Factors of fertility and infertility. *Psychoanalysis Inquiry*, 32 (3): 257–274.

Ferro, A. (2015). From Freud to Francis Bacon. *The Italian Psychoanalytic Annual*, 9: 175–187.

Ferro, A. and Civitarese, G. (2015). *The Analytic Field and its Transformations*. London: Karnac.

Flanders, S. (2015). On Piera Aulagnier's 'Birth of a Body, Origin of History'. *International Journal of Psychoanalysis*, 96 (5): 1403–1415.

Green, A. (1973). On negative capability: A critical review of W.R. Bion's Attention and Interpretation. *International Journal of Psychoanalysis*, 54: 115–119.

Grotstein, J.S. (2009). *'...But at the Same Time and on Another Level...'*, Vol. 1: *Psychoananlytic Theory and Technique in the Kleinian/Bionian Mode*. London: Karnac Books.

Lombardi, R. (2002). Primitive mental states and the body: A personal view of Armando B. Ferrari's Concrete Original Object. *International Journal of Psychoanalysis*, 83 (2): 363–381.

Lombardi, R. (2008). The body in the analytic session: Focusing on the body-mind link. *International Journal of Psychoanalysis*, 89 (1): 89–109.

Robert, P. (1984). *Le Petit Robert Dictionnnaire*. Paris: Le Robert.

Winnicott, D.W. (1958). The capacity to be alone. In *The Maturational Processes and the Facilitating Environment*. New York: International Universities Press. pp. 29–36.

Winnicott, D.W. (1966). Psycho-somatic illness in its positive and negative aspects. *International Journal of Psychoanalysis*, 47: 510–516.

Chapter 5

An invitation to think

Trauma, aporia[1] and the intersubjective
Field – A clinical example

David G. Power

Introduction

In describing Bion's contributions, Ogden (2008) states 'Bion's lifework as a psychoanalytic theorist was the formulation of a theory of thinking'. Beginning with his paper 'On arrogance' (1958), Bion emphasized the crucial role of the engaged, receptive and emotionally/psychically engaged other in the development of thinking, whether this other is the early caregiver or, later, the analyst. The most exciting and promising developments in current psychoanalytic theorizing and clinical application stem from Bion's discovery of the intersubjective nature of thinking, developments which have given us a fundamentally different orientation to psychoanalytic work, especially with those patients who do not fit easily into traditional nosological categories. The work of Winnicott fits here also in his emphasis on the fundamental importance of the real, external caregiving object in the development of a subjectively grounded and securely anchored self, including the sense of a body–mind connection that allows for a sense of inner experiential unity. Drawing in various degrees on these two thinkers, we enjoy what we can now understand as a truly *contemporary psychoanalysis*, international in nature and style, and recognizable in its emphasis on the deep, intersubjective and unconscious nature of psychic life. This contemporary psychoanalysis places heightened emphasis on the processual over content in the unfolding analytic hour, recognizes the foundational importance for mental life of a capacity for symbolization, and shows a renewed concern for theorizing the relationship of soma–psyche. Related to this latter interest, we now also see an attention to those aspects of mental life which are unrepresented (registered perhaps more in the body than the mind), and the challenges this non-representation places on clinical practice and on the practicing analyst. Among the many recent contributors in these areas I would mention Botella and Botella (2005), Brown (2011), Civitarese (2010), da Rocha Barros and da Rocha Barros (2011), Eshel (2013), Ferro (2009), Green (1999), Grotstein (2007), Levine (2012), Miller (2014), Mitrani (2001), Ogden (2005), and Roussillon (2011). My apologies to the many other important writers that space does not permit

DOI: 10.4324/9781003168034-5

mentioning. Each of these writers develop their ideas in conversation with Bion and Winnicott, drawing more or less heavily on one or both of them, conceptually and in sensibility.

It is within this larger fertile and creative dialogue that we can situate Bionian and post-Bionian Field Theory, developed and advanced by a small group of Italian analysts located in the north of Italy (primarily Pavia and Milan), among whom Antonino Ferro and Giuseppe Civitarese are perhaps the best known in North America. Unique to this group, and originally described in Ferro's initial conceptualizations, are the concepts of the 'Field' and of 'characters in the Field', an emphasis on the oneiric dimension of the analytic hour and an explicit emphasis on the goal of analysis as one of fostering the development of tools for thinking, a goal underwritten and promoted by the analyst's use of reverie and attention to a variety of transformational processes (i.e. transformation in dreaming, transformation in play, transformation in hallucinosis, etc.). The current volume and the essay I offer as part of it are testimony to the importance of this group's efforts in developing and extending many of the theoretical and clinical concerns enumerated above, and will hopefully expand further and develop these ideas in new and creative ways for those interested in them.

Trauma and the fracture of subjectivity

In the essay to follow I explore the deleterious effects of trauma on the capacity for thinking, a particular psychic state trauma creates in the personality and the relationship between this state and the symbolic forms available for representation of the trauma.[2] I present an extended clinical example illustrating movement from evacuative project identification toward greater capacity for symbolic expression of traumatic experience, a movement which I argue arises from the representational imperative activated in the patient, the analyst and in the Field itself (Levine, 2012) and which eventually leads to a dramatic, emotionally meaningful symbolic form (da Rocha Barros and da Rocha Barros, 2011) structured in the form of an aporia. This aporetic structure constitutes an important step in finding forms with which to think about experience which had previously remained enigmatic and irrepresentable and is a 'tool for thinking' par excellence for inviting further thought.

Trauma *qua* trauma is experience which must be endured but which cannot be psychically represented, and as such must be registered as something other than that which can be symbolized. Traumatic registrations are by their very nature closer to the soma than to the psyche and they persist as somatic events that point toward something but do not allow for this 'something' to be caught in a net of meanings, symbols, associations or dream narrations. They are carried as pointers toward 'undreamt dreams and interrupted cries' (Ogden, 2005), in need of and demanding, or as da Rocha Barros (2013) might prefer to say, 'inviting', an Other to 'think together' such that these registrations are afforded full gestation and birth as organized, psychically meaningful, symbolic forms. It is only then that 'thinking' in the Bionian sense can occur. It is this invitation to think that partly accounts for the origins and continual evolution of the intersubjective Field described in Bionian and post-Bionian Field Theory and is analogous to Ogden's concept of the intersubjective third. For this to occur in a fashion that generates its own continued evolution, expansion, and deepening this invitation must meet with an open and welcoming reception (a *projective identification welcoming object*) made known and available to the patient through its capacity for reverie and other transformational capacities (for instance, see Civitarese, 2015).

Without the occasion to meet such a psychically responsive and receptive Other, this invitation to think together is likely to wither and die (Roussillon, 2011), resulting in various alternative paths to expression other than ones that lead toward symbolization. Instead, these alternative paths lead toward varieties of acting out, discharge into the body (or soma), addictions and resort to sensory dominated modes of experience. To the extent that fantasy life is diminished (and in the case of trauma it is always diminished to a more or less significant extent), the psyche relies more heavily on splitting,[3] erasure, evacuation, foreclosure and denial. Action and simple discharge replace fantasy as a route of expression. If one were to think of this in terms of projective identification it appears as an increasing reliance on evacuative forms of projective identification over communicative forms. For patient and analyst, this shift in mode of participation naturally exerts heightened pressure on the Field itself (on the ability of the Field to contain, metabolize and transform an increased influx of beta elements) and according to the ethics of the Field, the burden of this pressure disproportionately falls to the analyst.

The difficulties with fantasy and representation, and the resulting modes of participation in the Field outlined above, signal the presence of a psyche traumatically dislocated from itself, unable to represent to and for itself, the cause and state of its alienation; a psyche structured around the uncanny, simultaneously present and absent, quality of traumatic experience. Structured in this way, traumatic experience is not envisioned and re-visioned (as in *nachtraglichkeit*). It cannot be captured and enfolded in a network of associations between and across levels of psychic functioning and so remains outside of the constant re-assessment of meanings that experience is otherwise subject to, and which affords an ongoing development, extension, elaboration and complexity of meanings (Green, 2000) and symbolic forms with which to represent them to oneself and others (da Rocha Barros and da Rocha Barros, 2011).

This alienation of the Self from its own experience is mirrored and doubled by alienation from the Other (more specifically, from the non-traumatized experience of the Other). Discussing the difficulties inherent in reading accounts of trauma, the literary critic Julian Wolfreys (2002), remarking on the radical disjunction that is existentially present between the traumatized psyche and the psyche of the concerned Other (read *analyst*), warns against a simple empathy or identification, and quoting Derrida suggests that the:

work of criticism becomes a matter of addressing the 'impossibility and necessity' of bearing witness to the 'unexperienced experience' (Derrida, 2000, p. 47), and it is through the structural gap, in that grammar of absence and loss, that the other comes to be heard.

(p. 133)

This same impossible necessity confronts and challenges the analyst invited to think by a traumatized patient.

Increasingly the reading of early Freud as emphasizing this return of repressed traumatic memory in action has been supplemented by a recognition that aspects of traumatic experience which never attained the status of organized, symbolically meaningful memory (and therefore susceptible to repression) may nonetheless be registered and subject to expression in forms of action or discharge that do not carry symbolic/fantasy meaning. These forms of registration suggest that the experience registered may never have been conscious, nor have had access to associational networks and elaboration in fantasy (Botella, 2014; Levine, 2012), either because they occurred developmentally prior to the psyche's maturing capacity for symbolization or they placed such demands on established capacities for symbolization that they overwhelmed them. Expressed in action, its 'meaning' therefore has less to do with content and more to do with pressure, expulsion or sheer discharge. Clinically, the demand on the analyst is less one of decoding a symbolic message and more one of assisting the patient in beginning to construct meanings, find words and create symbols that can begin to enfold the experience in processes leading toward narrative/fantasy elaborations (in the grammar of Bionian and post-Bionian Field Theory this enfolding process would be the generation of affective pictograms and their semiotic linkage in narrative derivations). In this sense, if the object recognizes the signal as such, its responsivity serves as a midwife to the action's evolution toward more symbolic forms of expression. This evolution affords the patient an opportunity to gather in and make sense of his experience (Winnicott, 1974) through access to alpha function, dreamwork, phantasy and insertion in associational networks. Seen from this perspective we have a 'theory of the object and of the manner in which the object subjectifies the self or enables the self to take on board the feeling of being a subject' (Roussillon, 2011, p. 171). This description of the process by which a subject becomes a subject is consistent with Freud's (1900, p. 615; 1915, p. 171) view, often referred to by Bion, that consciousness is the sense organ for the perception of psychic qualities, and accords with Williams's (2007) comment when describing disruptions in this process of subjectivation that 'in many seriously ill patients the mind remains an aspiration in what is essentially a reflexive existence [unless and until there] ... is a collaboration in the growth of a mind' (p. 401).

This radical dislocation of the subject from his/her own experience fractures a unified experience of personal history, obstructing any attempts at a subjectivation that leans toward a comprehensive and whole sense of oneself-in-the-world. Instead, an inarticulable gap is established in the psyche, on one side of which 'something happened' (the trace) while on the other side 'nothing happened' (the lack of mnemic representation). In contrast to the splitting that Freud (1940 [1938]) discussed, Roussillon (2011) describes this as a splitting that 'divides subjectivity into two parts, one of which is represented while the other is impossible to represent: it is, therefore, more a splitting done "to" the ego than one that is "of" the ego' (p. 13). From the standpoint of emotional truth, both and neither of these states of mind are true. This pairing of dual 'realities', each canceling, disputing, denying and erasing the other constitutes what in rhetorical and philosophical discussions has been called an 'aporia', and which has been explicitly applied to the study of trauma in literary criticism by Wolfreys (2002).[4] The concept has its origins in Greek philosophy, perhaps most prominently in Plato's recounting of the Socratic dialogues, and can be found as well in contemporary writings of post-structuralists, especially Derrida (2006).

The aporetic structure of traumatized subjectivity

The essential features of an aporia consist of: 1) an unresolvable logical contradiction posed by two diametrically negating propositions; 2) a radical state of doubt, confusion and impasse arising from the unresolvable nature of this contradiction.[5] As Socrates and Plato apparently understood, the logical disharmony at the heart of an aporia creates a reflected and parallel disharmony in the one who encounters it (an effect which the Socratic method relied on and honed to brilliance). An aporia engenders a fundamental imbalance in logic and, to the extent that the person(s) who encounter it are emotionally engaged with it and its consequences, imbalance in emotional stability as well. An aporia creates a flaw in one's experience of the world, and the 'rightness' of things that were previously relied on suddenly disappears, attended by distress and an irritable demand for resolution. The logical gap that is the aporia calls for some solution, for us to 'put things right again'. It is a call that is hard to ignore, yet not easy to answer. It compels us to think, to think again and think from many angles, much like turning an object in our fingers that looks vaguely familiar yet defies recognition.

> At first he did not know what [he thought he knew], and he does not know even now: but at any rate he thought he knew then, and confidently answered as though he knew, and was aware of no difficulty; whereas now he feels the difficulty he is in, and besides not knowing does not think he knows … [W]e have certainly given him some assistance, it would seem, towards finding out the truth of the matter: for now he will push on in the search gladly, as lacking knowledge; whereas then he would have been only too ready to suppose he was right …
>
> (Plato (1967), *Meno*, 84a–b)

The space that is held open by the conflicting ideas/experiences provokes the urge to fill it in and close the space and, were it possible to do so, promises a return to a state of psychic equilibrium and emotional certainty. Bion in his later writings warned against responding to this kind of urge, against reaching and against certainty, as does Ferro (2009). Yet this space, and the dissonance and tension that creates and maintains it, offers patient and analyst something more: an invitation to think:

> Now do you imagine he would have attempted to inquire or learn what he thought he knew, when he did not know it, until he had been reduced to the perplexity of realizing that he did not know, and had felt a craving to know? ... as a result of this perplexity, he will go on and discover something by joint inquiry with me ...
>
> (Plato (1967), *Meno*, 84c)

This power of the paradox that is an aporia breathes life and psychic vitality back into the sterile deadness of logic, 'fact' and the otherwise concretizing tyranny of a perception enslaved to the objective/external world, as well as to consciousness alone. Bion's distrust of the sensory world and preference for that which the analyst intuits can be understood as a recognition of this paradox, and it is obvious in Civitarese's (2015) discussion of transformations in hallucinosis as well. This same irritating, unsettling invitation to think is what the Socratic dialogues were about, a method designed to upend certainty, to bring disquiet and disharmony, and through this inducing of disturbance in that which is familiar offer the opportunity of a psychic space that invites new understanding. For this reason, the early Platonic dialogues are sometimes referred to as the 'aporetic dialogues'.

Is it by chance or style alone that Plato elects to describe the arrival of the aporia as a consequence of dialogue with an Other, an interpersonal if not intersubjective milieu? Or could it be that the presence of another inquiring mind, open to a discourse of curiosity and exploration, invites an environment in which fundamental contradictions of thought, perception and experience can find their initial expressive form?[6] Is this perhaps parallel to Roussillon's observation that the object is necessary for an encounter with one's experience which leads to deepening subjectivity? Can we assume that the dislocation of the self that is the sequela of trauma, and the 'radically discontinuous structure between self and other' (Wolfreys, 2002, p. 136) that it engenders, can only be recognized and encountered intersubjectively?

Symbolic forms and the imperative to represent

The work of da Rocha Barros (2013; da Rocha Barros and da Rocha Barros, 2011) is related to several of the points discussed so far. He directs our attention to the nature of the symbolic forms generated by the mind as a result of what he terms the *expressive function of the mind*, which he also connects to Levine's (2012) idea of a representational imperative. In da Rocha Barros's view, the mind searches for symbols to understand and to express (to oneself and others) its experience. These symbols perform a double function of both transmitting an emotional experience to someone and also representing it. When these two aspects are psychically conjoined then a mental representation is arrived at. However, da Rocha Barros (2013) suggests that the generating of a symbol does not necessarily imply that it serves the purpose of a mental representation since a symbolic form may remain as 'a first psychic inscription of an emotional experience' (p. 3). What then allows it to become a mental representation available for containment of emotion, experience and thought? 'For a symbolic form to assume the character of representation in the psychoanalytic sense of the term, it must be integrated in a subjectivity through a mental act of taking (it) over' (p. 3). Without this process of integrating the symbol into one's subjectivity, the symbolic form remains unusable for thought or self-reflection (it is only a proto-thought), and is usable only at the level of expressiveness, or as what da Rocha Barros calls a 'representation directed to someone' (not yet a truly mental representation). This act of expressiveness is the basis of communicative projective identification in his view, and it *evokes* in the mind of the other (assuming this mind is itself in contact with projective identification welcoming objects) a response that may ultimately lead to the subject's ability to integrate the symbolic form. Analytically this occurs because the evocation invites reverie, allows for psychic transformations to occur and for interpretations which allow the possibility of the patient integrating the symbol into his psychic world.

da Rocha Barros' description highlights a phenomenon frequently observed when working in areas closer to what has been referred to as 'the primordial mind' (Bion, 1976 Green, 1999; Scarfone, 2014). Here thought processes can appear to be built on a capacity for mental representation of experience as they are in the more highly organized and conflictually dominated areas of the mind. However, at this level of functioning what appear to the analyst to be mental representations that carry important symbolic content, and which can be analyzed as such, may not carry this meaning for the analysand. They may, and often are, not 'integrated into a subjectivity', and thus are serving as vehicles for evocation directed toward others, rather than as (yet) signaling their availability as carriers of symbolic meaning for the analysand. If misrecognized by the analyst they masquerade as harbingers of a capacity for thought but actually indicate experience which is still unrepresented or 'weakly represented' as Levine might tell us. In this state of masquerade, they act at best as proto-thoughts, capable through evocation of inviting analysand and analyst 'to think together'. At worse their misrecognition can lead to confusion, impasse or analysis at a superficial level.

Clinical material: Miriam

Miriam is a middle-aged woman who has been in treatment for several years. Chaos ruled her early family life. She and her siblings behaved wildly while suffering abandonment, loss and abuse. Grown, Miriam has prospered, and also suffered, by dint of her extraordinary work ethic. Her life is a non-stop blur of activity, tiring to imagine or listen to, and engendering ongoing complaints from the several men with whom she has had relationships.

In sessions, she recounts one situation after another, often full of apparent meanings and important themes, but shows little tolerance (or capacity) to reflect on them or consider their potential meaning or importance. That is to say, I hear many meanings in them but she seems oblivious, uninterested or incurious about the possible meanings of her experience. She seems lived by her experience rather than living it.

Efforts on my part to suggest or interpret or to connect events are typically met with dismissal, incredulity and denigration. I find her reactions disorienting, confusing and at times annoying. Each time I try to psychologically or emotionally 'connect' with her I feel blocked out, ignored, dismissed and often end up feeling stupid or ashamed for having made the effort. For instance, she has frequently made comments that she 'can't believe she may never be pregnant' but if I comment about a wish to have a child she reacts loudly that she has no interest in children and would never want to be a mother. So I take her reactions as a bit of supervision, an 'analytic GPS signal' (Levine, 2015, p. 461), telling me that this comment is too direct (too saturated), too emotionally 'hot', and therefore intolerable and disturbing. So a bit later I venture several less saturated comments, suggesting perhaps that she 'wishes for something more inside herself', or on another occasion that she 'wishes that together with someone she might create something more in her life', trying in this way to offer something I feel will be less saturated, less full of specific meaning and which might allow her to engage with it and enter a verbal 'Squiggle Game'. But each time she reacts with equal disdain, leaving me to feel I can never quite get it right. Like in the fairy tale of the Three Bears, my analytic 'porridge' seems always to be the wrong temperature.

Not infrequently these outbursts of hers leave me feeling humiliated. I stress this reaction of mine because, though I have a theory that helps me to 'understand' them, my discomfort serves to indicate an immersion in the intersubjective Field that has, and is, developing between us. The key importance of this lies in the fact that our *seeming* inability to make emotional/ subjective contact with each other is actually a *beginning form of contact*, as long as it can eventually become an 'analytic object', and therefore an object of analytic interest and curiosity in itself (Bergstein, 2015; Eaton, 2011).

Throughout our work together Miriam has characteristically dismissed almost all feelings, her own or mine, as 'sentimental', 'complaining' or otherwise mawkish, while at the same time complaining that her boyfriends don't regard her feelings or needs enough, and instead are 'numb' emotionally. She describes her father as also having had a particular hatred toward any feeling or emotional need. This latter description often calls to my mind a comment of Bion's that it is only a short step from hating emotions to hating life itself (Bion, 1959).

For several years we had been meeting three times per week with Miriam choosing to sit up during her treatment. Prior to the session I am about to describe, Miriam had dropped her Friday sessions because of a new job that required her to work longer hours. At our next session Miriam sat down, scrutinized me with a scowling, accusatory expression and said, 'You are pre-occupied!' Her tone was scolding and withering in its disapproval. Not aware of being preoccupied, I was taken aback by her vehemence. Actually, I had been thinking about our last session and appreciating again the disorienting effect she often has on me. But we ended in better contact in her previous visit and I was unprepared for this beginning to our session.

Surprised by Miriam's opening remark I was speechless. I felt stunned, as if I had been suddenly accosted. She went on to talk about feeling fat, her frustration shopping for a dress for a friend's wedding, her dislike of dressing up and her preference for wearing 'hand-me-down', used clothes. At this point I began to think of my own childhood dislike of 'inheriting' things from my older brother and wondered if her preference for used clothes might be an attempt to disown feelings of unimportance and humiliation at being the youngest child, and youngest of several girls, in a large family, and in the transference of being no longer of much importance to me. *(Noticing my thoughts and reactions, I tried to use them to understand their meaning in the here-and-now of the session, assuming from the vertex of the Field that everything in the hour refers to the hour itself, even if the overt references are to people or events outside the hour. For instance, the wedding and the feelings about dressing up or dressing down can be heard as the initial 'casting of characters in the Field', the session's early 'affective holograms'* (Ferro, 2009). *Listened to in this way these 'characters' vivify and help give initial narrative form to the beginning emotional concerns of our coming together in the session).*

Miriam continued, referring to her older sister 'who is tall, beautiful and can wear anything' and recalls growing up too poor to wear stylish clothes in a wealthy suburban high school. She was annoyed, sarcastic and dismissive. Suddenly there was a loud noise in the waiting room, which I share with another analyst. Late for an appointment, another patient had entered the waiting room talking loudly on a cell phone. Calling out to my suitemate, a tall, thin woman who dresses stylishly, he apologizes for his lateness. While exchanging greetings he continues talking loudly to her as they walk past my office door toward her office. Suddenly they fall quiet.

I find myself quite distracted and psychically contaminated by this intrusion. The feeling I noticed at the beginning of the hour, of being suddenly accosted and assaulted, threatens to overtake me again. At the corner of my awareness I noticed that I imagine my suitemate as Miriam's sister, arriving home from a date. Then I think of humiliation and recall a 'funny thought' Miriam once shared about the possibility that my suitemate might be my daughter.

Miriam says angrily, 'I hate that woman, and I think you hate her too'. Without thinking I say, 'I hate the noise'. I feel completely off-guard by the suddenness of this intrusion in my previously totally quiet office and feel very guilty and apologetic that I could not prevent this from happening and disturbing my analysand. Looking back on this moment, I now also think that I unconsciously 'protected' my suitemate, like any good father might do, by focusing my comment on the noise and deflecting my anger off of her, in that way declining Miriam's offer to join with her in targeting my suitemate (her sister and my preferred daughter in the transference).

I was aware at this point of thinking another 'child' has noisily arrived, just as Miriam and I had begun to settle back in together and the accusatory atmosphere that began the session was waning. Slight feelings of humiliation and shame lingered on the edges of my awareness, connected to feelings that with such a noisy office, I was an impostor as an analyst. *(Reflecting on this later I recognized how readily I dressed myself in 'hand-me-down clothes' and wrestled with the humiliation of being a pretender 'dressed' in analyst's clothing. External events (here, the arrival of my suitemate's noisy patient) can quickly become part of the Field and the 'ongoing dream of the session').*

Miriam answered, 'I bet they got quiet because she remembered that Dr. Power told her to be quiet and it's the only thing he has really asked of her!' I was again startled by her response and wondered how I should understand it. Unsure of myself, I felt diminished in my sense of being a 'real' analyst because of Miriam's beginning accusation, then followed by my inability to offer her a quiet and secure space. Yet she suddenly seemed to find me strong, in charge, comfortingly secure and on her side. Was she now feeling safer because I did not join her in criticizing my roommate and felt I would be less likely to be critical of her?

To my relief she then returned to the plans for the weekend wedding. 'That anorexic woman I told you about who is so pretty is going to be there. Kevin (Miriam's boyfriend) told me that I shouldn't worry about her, that she is not his type. So that makes it a little better'. I heard this as confirming my previous thoughts that she was feeling more settled with me now and felt that my interest was with her. *(The appearance of the character of 'Kevin' at this moment who reassures her 'not to worry about another woman' suggests that somehow Miriam was feeling comforted, more accepted and emotionally secure now together with me. From this listening vertex, characters enter the Field like actors entering onto a stage in order to exemplify, embody and give expression to emotions as they evolve and transform as the session unfolds. Thus the Field offers us an additional listening perspective – one that constantly orients and re-orients us toward Miriam's inner life, the evolution of her emotions and the developing state of her capacity to represent it to herself and to others, thus allowing her to think about herself and her experience).*

In response to Miriam's comment 'Kevin told me not to worry about her, she's not my type, so that makes it a little better', I said 'I can understand why you are so upset about your weight and finding just the right dress. When you are with your man it's important to feel attractive and that you hold his attention and don't feel you are a "hand-me-down"'. *(I said this in hopes of addressing what I felt was her unexpressed shame that she is second-class for me compared to my suitemate. Even though I had begun to think that Miriam felt less persecuted in my presence and that*

*our contact was more collaborative – that is, that we were more of a
'couple' emotionally working productively together. Based on the way the
hour had begun and on past experience I was reluctant, nonetheless, to offer
too saturated a comment. So I kept my remark open as to its referents, both
in terms of the 'man' and the 'holding his attention' to which I was referring. In this way I hoped to give her as much psychological room as possible
from which to hear my meanings and/or create her own).*

She then talked about confronting her boyfriend over hitting his children. She
worries it might end the relationship but instead he listened to her and said he
would think about what she said. Afterward he asked her to accompany him to
visit a friend whose wife has just had a baby. *(I took this as a communication from
the Field that Miriam heard my comment and felt relieved by it. I imagined myself
as the boyfriend who needed to be confronted for mistreating his children, as
Miriam confronted me at the beginning of the session. I then imagined her
experiencing the sudden loud noise in the waiting room as a child might when
suddenly struck by a parent. I thought she might fear that our relationship could
suddenly erupt in violence, emotionally or physically, and finds my response
instead to be an invitation to engage in creative emotional work together. That is,
rather than our emotional contact being violent and destructive, it could be fertile
and constructive. In this series of thoughts I was 'dreaming the session' and by
doing so also 'dreaming the patient into life' – that is, drawing upon my emotionally laden, subjective immersion in the session with Miriam to construct, attribute
and infer meaning to Miriam's and my experience. This was an attempt to address
and to redress Miriam's limitations in providing this function for herself. The goal
was to assist Miriam in expanding these capacities in herself, safeguarded by my
efforts to attend continuously to how Miriam experiences my presence and comments. It is the analyst's ongoing responsibility to participate in the Field while
constantly listening for and responding to signals from it. This is why listening,
from within the Field, to reactions to interventions in the Field is so important).*

Continuing her story of confronting Kevin, his surprising reaction and his
invitation to visit the new parents together, Miriam said, 'I couldn't understand
why he still wanted to do that with me after what I said, but he seemed fine with
it. So, we went to see them and he held the baby. It is really something to see him
with a baby – he has these big hands and he really knows how to hold a baby,
totally confident and gentle, he's had a lot of practice I guess'.

I responded that I thought 'this would make a baby feel very safe and
secure and that a couple would feel confident having a baby if they knew they
could rely on each other to know how to care for it'. I said this because I
heard her communication as referring to young and tender feelings that
needed to be given birth, and which require strong hands to hold and keep
safe. She seemed to be venturing a surprised recognition (and hope) that this
birth might be possible in our relationship. *(I am not implying she was aware
that her thoughts and feelings refer directly to us. I responded the way I did
because I thought she was still not ready to hear a comment that was too*

saturated, as a straightforward transference comment would have been. Instead I wanted my comment to remain rather general and unspecific as to its referent, in order that her thinking could have as much room as possible to expand and develop. I continued to feel there was a very fragile line for her between emotional contact which was experienced as secure, safe and generative and contact which was frightening, violent and destructive).

She then started to tell me about an incident with Kevin's 7-year-old son, Jamie. 'The kids seemed really glad to see me, which really surprises me. I felt kind of guilty about it because I don't want to act like I am their mother. The kids get into it and get really materialistic but what they really want is to spend time with their dad and be very physical – you know, rough-housing. I'm not sure he understands this'. I heard this as an expression of her yearning for a contact with me in the transference that she could feel in a more psychologically tangible way and her belief that I am deaf to this wish. *(Continuing to listen from the perspective of the Field I tried to de-concretize this story and began to wonder if I was now too unsaturated in my comments. Did she want more 'roughhousing' together – meaning more direct, saturated 'give and take' that might resemble more traditional transference interpretations? There was now also the return of the theme of 'motherhood' and her complicated yearnings for, and warded off wishes to have, children).*

'Then I did a totally strange and crazy thing – I can't believe it and can't understand why I did it. I had kept a dried leaf on the dashboard of my car for months – I liked the way it looked all dried and curled up. Kevin knew this and one day it went missing and he said he had thrown it out the window. He hadn't but had hidden it in his pocket instead – he was teasing me'.

Miriam continued, 'So I found another leaf and replaced it. But this day I said to Jamie "Let's have a contest. I'll give you this leaf to put in this box and if you can keep it safe and give it back to me in a week then I'll give you a reward!" So, I got a small piece of wood and carved his name in it. I asked him if he knew his last name because I don't know if seven-year-olds normally know their last names or not. And his father overheard us and kept saying to him "Yes, but do you know how to spell it?" in an intimidating and threatening way'. *(Hearing this vignette as reflecting yet another evolution in her experience of contact with me, I noticed how quickly the 'gentle man with the big hands' became taunting and teasing. I imagined the possible danger Miriam might feel giving over to me any of the 'baby feelings' she seemed earlier to hope I might hold securely. I think emotional closeness and contact with a man is very frightening and unpredictable for Miriam, constantly and suddenly shifting between her yearnings and hopes for more of it and her fears that closeness would suddenly erupt into taunting, intimidation and violence. This latter fragility seemed to confirm my reluctance to 'rough-house' with her by offering too direct and saturated comments. Yet in another way I wonder if by remaining cautiously unsaturated in my comments I am refusing to see what is in plain sight – her wish to be 'owned' by a parent (knowing her last name), her depressed state that this need goes unrecognized and the taunting cruelty this represents to her. Listened to in this way, the dried, curled up leaf she places on her dashboard for anyone to see is another character, and gives narrative life to her dysphoric longings to be attached to me more firmly – and the character of Kevin becomes an affective hologram for the person who teases her and her disappointed longings, by cruelly taking them and seeming to discard them as useless).*

Miriam continued with her story. 'I carved his first and last name in the wood and then shellacked it several times, and when he gave me the leaf back I gave it to him as a gift'. *(Deciding to offer something more saturated, but still keeping it outside the immediate here-and-now of our relationship)* I said, 'Perhaps you understood how Jamie felt, confused about what was happening with his parents and feeling very lost, like you felt when you were little and your parents split up. You want to claim Jamie from these two adults but feel guilty about this wish. I think you want to make sure both of you know what his name is – who he belongs to'. *(When she seemed to tolerate this comment without objecting, I added)* 'I think you also feel lost and thrown away yourself like the leaf in the car, and not sure who you belong to. You feel discarded by Kevin like you do by your father'.

Miriam listened quietly to all that I said, and so I offered something quite saturated and specific to our relationship and said 'Maybe you feel painfully discarded here (with me) as well and that's why you think I was preoccupied at the beginning of the hour. You feel I was elsewhere in my mind'.

To my surprise she seemed to experience these comments with relief, nodding and looking away as if full of feeling. This reaction was very unusual because she typically objected strongly and protested loudly against any comments about our relationship, saying some version of 'we don't have a relationship' or 'I don't have any feelings about you' or 'I don't need you'.

But this time instead of objecting she says softly, 'My father acts like he doesn't even have any children'. I felt something release inside of me with this statement, as if I had been holding a muscular tension I was not aware of but now no longer needed to hold.

I respond, 'It's a terrible thing to be the daughter of a father who has no children', and she bursts out crying, continuing crying until the session ended. She had never wept like this before with me, and in fact has never cried at all in a session.

Unlike the beginning of the session I felt we ended the hour in good contact. Perhaps because of this I began to notice some reluctance to experience the keenness of her sense of rejection by me despite having commented on it. I further realized that I had not spoken directly to her of the connection between her feeling discarded and the dropped session. Nor had I connected any of this with the manner in which she denigrates the meaningfulness of our relationship.

I began to notice in myself the glimmerings of shame stemming from what I experienced as Miriam's rejection of me (by insisting on dropping a session and frequently proclaiming that we did not have a relationship). Although she was the leaf her father/boyfriend/analyst was throwing away, so also was I being thrown away by her as I suspect she felt I was throwing her away by allowing her to drop the session. This was also another meaning of the abuse of the children – we were in a relationship in which people who should care for each other punish and persecute each other instead.

I had been aware of the dropped session, but it existed in my mind as a fact without immediate emotional valence during most of the session. As I began to reflect on this I remembered the feelings of shame and humiliation connected to being an 'imposter analyst' that I had noticed arising in myself earlier in the session. When Miriam initially accused me of being preoccupied I had not made the obvious connection to the missed session – so in fact I was preoccupied (mentally occupied with something other than Miriam and our missed time together). I was instead thinking of the good contact with which we had ended our last meeting. In this way I was preoccupied with, and anticipating the arrival of, the Miriam of the last session and not awaiting the Miriam who would arrive for the current day's session (Bion, 2013 [1967]). This preoccupation with the Miriam of yesterday characterized the obstructed quality of our contact, and paradoxically marked both the limit of our receptivity toward each other and simultaneously served as the opportunity for its transformation over the course of the session.

Discussion

I will now trace the evolution, deepening and expansion in the capacities of the Field to contain, tolerate, engender and inspire forms of expression and thought during the course of the hour, eventuating in the arrival of an aporia that captures in its simple distillation the complexities of Miriam's traumatic experience. I argue that in its arrival it both announces the fruit of our 'thinking together' and carries within its form the challenge of, and opportunity for, further thinking together, if its enigmatic, paradoxical tension is sustained.

I stand accused from the outset of 'being preoccupied' and this accusation hits me like a blow against which I have to struggle to maintain my emotional and psychic balance and in the face of which I 'forget' the missed session. This 'communication' from Miriam is in the form of an evacuative projective communication and its expressive value is in its evocation in me of a state of shame and abasement ('I am an imposter analyst') with which I then have to struggle to consciously recognize, contain and work with in reverie. Because of the intensity of Miriam's charge and the manner in which it was abruptly made and then seemingly abandoned (she showed no ability to discuss and explore it), it appears to be little more than an expulsion of something bothersome and unwanted, an irritable discharge that did not carry much in the way of symbolic meaning for her. Had I been able to connect her comment to the missed session I doubt she would have seen a connection and might instead have been simply perplexed, and become denigrating and dismissive. This type of engagement is less an invitation to think together and more of a potential opportunity to do so, as it places most of the burden on the analyst. Its form signals Miriam's desperate need for a receptive, engaged other who can provide containment in the form of reverie and initial representation.[7]

The shame and humiliation I experienced in the face of Miriam's accusation prompted in me a surprising (to me) string of memories about my own experiences as a child in a large family and a growing, and more explicit for me, appreciation of the sense of unimportance I attributed to my status as recipient of my brother's used and no longer needed clothing. This memory provided me with a beginning relief from the shame I felt and allowed me to feel I was beginning to regain my mind and imaginal capacities, partly because it provided a third reference (memories of my childhood and specifically my sibling relationship) which decreased the immediate intensity I experienced upon receiving Miriam's projective assault. Yet the recall of my own experience at being diminished as a child of 'lesser importance' allowed me to begin to de-concretize the exchange and begin to make a subjective experience into an object of analytic curiosity. I was then able to begin absorbing and transforming the experience, a process expressed through my constructing an imagined image of Miriam's experience. Thus the initial accusatory exchange, an example of her typical aggressive and dismissive attitude toward me, enacted both an obstructive link to the object (the evacuation) and offered the possibility of this traumatic experience being received and transformed by the object through reverie (its communicative function). As both Bergstein (2015) and Eaton (2011) have written, an attack on linking in the clinical setting also tells the story of an early infantile emotional catastrophe and in doing so offers a moment for its beginning transformation.

As I was beginning to regain my balance in the session there is the noisy arrival of my suitemate's male patient, disorienting me again with this sudden feeling of being assaulted and accosted. I imagined the arrival of one of Miriam's many older siblings, coming home from a date with her boyfriend. Spontaneously, Miriam shared a fantasy that the other 'couple' in the suite had gotten quiet because I had spoken to my suitemate in the past and asked them to be quiet, the 'only thing you ever asked them'. I was conscious of my annoyance, a reaction to again feeling plunged into inner confusion and humiliation over being an inadequate analyst. I commented abruptly and without any contemplation that I 'hated the noise', a response I understood retroactively as a paternal urge to protect my suitemate from criticism and to resist 'siding' with Miriam in her obvious contempt for her. Miriam returned to her discussion of the upcoming wedding and specifically her fear that an 'anorexic woman' would be there and prove more attractive to her boyfriend than would Miriam. She then reported her relief at her boyfriend's reassurance that this other woman 'is not his type'.

I think at this point I was finally able to get past the session's repeated chaotic disruptions and their effect on me to begin to dream the session. I was able to shift once again (or finally) and to register the arrival of several characters in the form of the boyfriend, the anorexic woman threatening to compete for his attention and the wedding. The interruption itself was now available for dreaming as well, a good illustration of how an actual event quickly becomes enfolded into the ongoing dream of the session. From the vertex of the session and the dream of the hour, we moved toward a still unsaturated but somewhat more discernible (to me) 'consideration' of our own readiness to marry, that is to say, our availability for joint communion. Although I could recognize it only in retrospect, the initial accusation of 'you are preoccupied' can be seen as a distressed call for my availability. It was a noisy harbinger of what was now evolving as our emotional narrative of the session, and the 'preference' for hand-me-down clothes as a characterization of herself as diminished and unnoticeable. From this retrospective look, Miriam's fantasy that I had told my suitemate to be quiet can be understood as a request to me to silence distractions (other women, other children, other preoccupations) and turn my attention to her. (I stress again that these are retrospective understandings, or perhaps we can say retrospective dreams of the session.)

At this point in the session the initial evacuative projective identification has been contained and transformed. A process of thinking and inviting thinking is developing in the Field, and the qualities of the Field are increasingly more communicative and less evacuative. Careful attention to the saturation level of my comments supports and fosters this evolution. The space which is now opening in our way of relating to each other is illustrated by, and allows for, a greater shift toward reverie, freedom to associate, intrusions of stray and sudden thoughts, flashes of images or somatic reactions. Characters are being generated, and narrations initiated, inviting us to think together (dream), although the forms generated and offered are asymmetrically meaningful. That is to say, characters and narrative threads imply and embody representational forms that are more de-concretized, more abstract, and more associatively rich for me than they are for Miriam.

Calmer now, I commented in a very unsaturated way, connecting several of Miriam's references to weight, clothing and the fear of other women making noises that distract men to a wish to feel confident and assured that she can 'hold the attention of her man'. My phrasing is purposely vague in its referent so as to allow Miriam to respond as freely as possible and without the constraints that burden an explicit transference comment. The form of my comment calls for and 'carries' an invitation to think, an invitation to join me in thinking together about our emotional situation (the possibility of our intersubjective marriage and its potential fertility). But it does so in a manner which leaves open the nature of our relationship, its exact place in our dialogue, and where the limits to its representation may lie.

In the past Miriam may have responded by denigrating and dismissing my empathic suggestion that she might feel insecure (despite having voiced it herself) but instead she shared new material and revealed new anxieties, specifically her fears at confronting her boyfriend over his physical violence and a gentle and caregiving side of him that she had not described before and which seemed to surprise her. From a Field perspective this seemed to confirm my earlier comment. There now seemed to be a willingness and capacity to dream the possibility of a closeness and intimacy without violence, and of the possibility of turning a baby aspect of herself (another character) over to a man for nurturance and caretaking. The arrival of the character of a man who is both strong, nurturant, safe and whose caregiving was focused on her was completely unanticipated by me, and was unprecedented in her telling of her history, contemporary social life or inter-actions with me. Her stated fear of confronting her boyfriend over hitting his children, my feeling of being physically assaulted by her accusation and my reveries about the noisy patient being experienced as a frightening intruder by a child version of my patient all indexed the psychic work she had accom-plished by now casting her boyfriend as a character embodying nurturance, security and physical safety. From the vertex of the Field, this amounted to a transformation in that moment of her emotional experience of me and of us, a representation of us and of herself as in a relationship of care, fertility, safety and dependence.

Responding to the birth of this image (the casting of this character), I emphasized the safety a baby would feel and the confidence a couple would have knowing they could rely on each other to care for the baby. This again was a purposely unsatu-rated comment meant to underscore the emotional implications of her image while leaving her ample room to continue 'thinking' about it.

Miriam responded by recounting a long, complicated story that presented her boyfriend now as a teasing, playful man whose humor seemed to hint at sadistic enjoyment and whom she described in a way that seemed intimidat-ing, demanding and dominating toward his son. Themes of loss and aban-donment, confusion over what one's name was and what family one belonged to, and of the impermanence of familial connection emerged. I was struck by the transformation of the boyfriend character from strength, kindness and security into a menacing, teasing and dominating character. A deep anxiety permeated the story which Miriam tried to 'solve' by making a nameplate, expressing what seemed to be a very concrete way of reassuring herself that identity and family connection could be permanently and objectively estab-lished. The character of the dead leaf, preserved and kept on her dashboard until her boyfriend removed it, suggested an underlying sadness and depres-sion which though in plain sight went unappreciated and disappeared. The 'game' her boyfriend played by taking the leaf perhaps signifying a mocking, intentionally dismissive refusal to recognize the pain it represented.

In response to what I experienced as a deeply moving story I offered a number of quite specific and saturated comments linking together her fears of not belonging, the confusion and chaos of feeling lost, untethered and forgotten about in her primary relationships, and a specific experience of feeling discarded by me. And I linked this last comment to her accusation that I was preoccupied. In doing so I was far more saturated and direct than I had previously been in the session but I felt there had been a building emotional intensity, thematic clarity and deepening contact and that my comments were little more than overt recognition of the emotional warp and woof that constituted our thinking together in the session. Miriam seemed to confirm this when, instead of dismissing my comment that she felt discarded by me, responded instead by saying that her father acted as if he had no children, a statement filled with uncharacteristic resignation and sadness.

My final comment to Miriam came to me without any conscious consideration whatsoever, and in fact I 'heard' it simultaneously with her, speaking the words without first thinking them. It seemed to simply arrive, all of a piece with the hour and with her statement that her father acted as if he had no children. From a Field perspective my comment was a joint creation and evolved out of the Field itself. If everything is 'in and from the Field' then the phrase 'my final comment' is only an artifact of speech. It would be more accurate, although clumsier, to say 'in that particular moment I gave voice to this comment arising from the Field'.

Although my comment remained very close to hers, my use of the phrase 'a terrible thing' made more palpable to both of us the deep pain of the existential predicament with which she was forced to live. In addition, the slight shift in phrasing from 'my father' to her 'being a daughter of a father ...' may have served to draw her and my attention more clearly to the emotionally disorienting, logically inconsistent and therefore destabilizing aporetic structure of her experience.

The session demonstrates Miriam's ability to use a containing object to arrive at a moment where she can bear moving closer to her emotional truth (Levine, 2010) and learn from it, thereby moving closer to her own internal world. This lessening of her need for evacuation rested on my tolerance for being a projective identification welcoming object. And it rested as well on our gradual and joint success in creating an intersubjective Field in which the qualities of dreaming and reverie became ascendant over mere evacuation. This intersubjective collaboration allowed us to arrive at a succinct, emotionally evocative image (a beginning mental representation), born of the fertility of the Field, that she was 'a daughter of a father who had no children'. There was an immediacy and aliveness to this moment that sprung from its capacity to serve as a condensation of her experience, connecting many psychic and emotional layers and helping her move from experience that was unfelt to experience that was suddenly felt.

The sudden emergence of intense sadness and loss, marked by Miriam's weeping at the session's close, suggests it was a moment of *epiphanic intensity* (da Rocha Barros, 2013) when the expressive character of the symbol vivifies the imagined form, allowing for a perception 'of a meaning through sudden intuition which is at the same time simple and shocking' (p. 9). Miriam was able to further integrate into her subjectivity what she had experienced but not fully known, a moment when a mental representation of her experience became available. I believe my own sudden experience of relief mirrored this epiphanic intensity and signaled as well my deepening capacity to serve in that moment as a projective identification welcoming object. The suddenness and spontaneity of the arrival in my mind of the realization I offered Miriam (the essential horror of being the daughter of a father who has no children) was our 'epiphany' for the session, an epiphany we arrived at conjointly. The suddenness of its realization, although carrying with it emotional relief and release, had a vitalizing and enlivening feel to it, as if Miriam and I, as well as our relationship, had suddenly been given a new birth. This experience of aliveness is reminiscent of Scarfone's (2014) metaphor of the oculus and the vitality that emerges from the unknown that energizes but evades complete representation. It is a moment of 'lived experience instead of a mere evocation' (pp. 4–5).

The invitation of the aporia

da Rocha Barros (2013) says rather poetically, 'an image or symbolic form thinks and invites the interlocutor who sees it to think together' (p. 3). An aporia, by virtue of its structure, offers a particularly strong invitation in this regard. In Miriam's case the recognition that she 'was the daughter of a father who had no children' provided an initial, quite succinct representation of her experience as at once being in a relational structure explicitly established and sanctioned culturally, socially and psychically, while simultaneously having this experience denied, erased and negated. The first reality (being the daughter of a father) is an exoteric one, based on everyday external reality and common understanding, while the second, negated reality is an esoteric one, private and known-from-within. The space that lies in between these two 'realities' outlines and delimits the traumatic experience which Miriam (and now me) confronted. Like an aporia that contrasts logically contradictory postulates and thereby threatens any security built on simple rationality alone, this representation of her reality (and even the word 'reality' inaccurately portrays a unitary experience) provides a constant threat to the identity she consciously maintained in the face of her traumatic experience, a quite rigid but therefore fragile adaptation maintained by exiling much of her emotional life. As she and I were able to jointly arrive at a more complexly nuanced statement of her father's relationship to her, the impact of her father's profound lack of emotional investment in being a father (he has no children) was laid bare, and exposed its existential threat to her; the negation of her identity as a 'daughter to her father'. In this way the lack of investment by the object in its role *vis-à-vis* the subject assaults the subject's narcissistic investment at the level of identity/integrity. This is so because every object representation is *ipso facto*, and simultaneously, a self-representation (Botella and Botella, 2005).

Although tumultuous, the instability that accompanied Miriam's fuller recognition of her emotional dilemma in relationship to her father announced a greater emotional capacity and presented an opportunity for creative and vitalizing psychic work, work that further invited the two of us to 'think together'. Describing the creative potential (that is, not tied entirely to objective fact) of what they call 'negative higher unities', the Botellas (2005, p. 28) describe how the *addad*[8] 'easily destabilize preconscious formations and give rise to a withdrawal of investment from the realm of representation … word presentations are erased, making way for hallucinatory tendencies' (p. 25). Civitarese (2015) has similarly described this process (from the analyst's perspective) in this way: 'what seems evident from the point of view of the senses or a certain theoretical system can easily obstruct the analyst's ability to perceive something new, and hence to be receptive to the facts of the analysis' (p. 1100). The aporetic realization which culminates this hour with Miriam is made possible by a joint 'blinding' of ourselves to the material reality of fatherhood in order to 'see the hallucinated' reality that she is the daughter of a father without children. This blinding can occur because at this moment in the hour the Field's oneiric qualities have evolved so as to foster a suspension of material reality in the service of recognizing another, psychic reality. This is her emotional reality, the esoteric reality, out of contact with which leaves her only a sterile, emotionally denuded reality of a 'father'. This latter was the 'solution' to the trauma, a solution now destabilized in the effort toward growth.

What emotional future is implied by arriving at a logic which itself is illogical and irreconcilable? How does one proceed in the face of it? Does 'proceed' even have a meaning, and if so, what meaning, in the face of it? We can begin to respond to this interrogation by noting the distance traversed in the hour, a distance that marks a movement from expulsion/short circuiting of thought to a beginning contemplation freighted with sadness and loss. This movement is made possible and substantially underwritten by the mutually elicited, and responded to, invitations to think (as well as the initial evacuative 'opportunity to think'), themselves taking several evolving forms along the trajectory from the horizon to their arrival at the hour's close. One response to the questions posed above may be simply 'proceed as we have proceeded'. Would this not be what Bion's concept of 'faith' might imply?

Derrida (2006) approaches this question in his monograph on *Aporias* and argues for the necessity of *experiencing* it rather than attempting to resolve it:

> What if the exoteric aporia therefore remained in a certain way irreducible, calling for an endurance, or shall we say an experience other than that consisting in opposing from both sides of an indivisible line, an other concept, a non-vulgar concept, to the so-called vulgar concept? … And is it an issue of an *either/or*? Can one speak – and if so, in what sense – *of an experience of the aporia?* An experience *of the aporia as such?*
>
> (pp. 14–15)

Rather than a solution to the unsolvable, Derrida's call for experiencing derides solution itself[9] and declares that experiencing is 'neither stopping [at the impasse] nor overcoming it' (p. 32). What then is left to us? What way forward is there – or perhaps better stated, from where does further evolution arise?

If there is an analytic answer to this challenge, it must be an intersubjective one, one that draws on a phenomenology that recognizes both unshared and shared experience, and the complicated manner in which they commingle and create each other. One is reminded here of Eshel's (2013) work with severely traumatized patients and a series of case reports wherein she details her subjectively excruciating psychic engagement with a patient deeply entrenched in a sadomasochistic world. Striking though her capacity for sustained deep engagement is, this engagement leads her ineluctably to a moment where she appears to surrender her capacity for understanding and contact, only to discover at this moment of despair an experience of being taken over by a vision which, somewhat alien in nature, allowed her to access a level of communion with her patient's experience which had eluded her to that point.[10] From a Field perspective experiences like this (rather than solutions), highlight the importance of the Field's aspiration toward unison and the power of such experience midwifing an understanding distinctly different from, and more transformative than, that which arrives from 'the outside' (O vectoring toward K, rather than K vectoring toward O) (Civitarese, 2015; Ferro, 2009, 2012). In these moments, the impasse of the aporia is encountered not simply by the patient but also more directly by the analyst; in Eshel's felicitous phrase, by 'withnessing', an intersubjective valence toward joining that fosters and enables a claiming for the first time of traumatic experience by the ego (that which happened to the subject but was not experienced by the subject due to immaturity of the ego and/or an excessiveness of stimulation). Eshel's appreciation for Winnicott's (1974) insights is made obvious here. Crucial in this process are the analyst's porosity, permeability and receptiveness (Civitarese, 2015; Miller, 2014) which make the analyst available to partially take on the burden of the patient's experience (Grotstein, 2007) without collapsing entirely the un-traversable difference between the two (that is, respecting the fundamental singularity of traumatic experience). Just as Derrida (2006) argues for a logic of the aporia that 'does not oppose figures to each other, but instead installs the haunting of the one in the other' (p. 20), the same can be said about the patient's and the analyst's experience. A willingness to be haunted may be a fundamental obligation of the analyst and of a Field capable of engaging and containing traumatic experience. From this point of view, my being 'preoccupied' at the beginning of the session with Miriam may have been my unconscious effort to refuse a 'haunting', or in Civitarese's (2015) view my insisting on an emotionally denuded view of our relationship (transformation in hallucinosis) because it relied on a now idealized view of our last session rather than an openness and receptivity to the immediate moment.

The arrival in our discourse of a statement capturing Miriam's emotional dilemma invites (compels) further thinking because it allows for:

hidden meanings that being absent, are kept in suspension, therefore in a potential state. This absence of meaning does not reduce itself to the mere concealment of a presence: it is a state of suspension, an absent reference or even a discontinuity, which constantly leads the psyche to having to broaden its means of representation. This constitutes a response to an absence permanently present, of a discontinuity never to be overcome.

(da Rocha Barros, 2013, p. 14)

At the end of the hour there is a deepening emotional atmosphere apparent in Miriam's palpable sadness as well as my sense of physical release. What does this shift in mood imply for the further work of representation? If, as was suggested earlier, the object representation is always also a self-representation (a self-representation/object representation), then her father's perceived lack of investment in his role as father to her means for Miriam a concomitant and catastrophic lack of investment in herself, or said otherwise, an intolerable lack of investment in a narcissistically stabilizing self-representation/object representation. The echoes of this lack of investment can be heard in her insistent statements to me that 'we don't have a relationship' and her haughty, contemptuous dismissal of feelings, her own and mine. The aporia succinctly captured both her attempt to deny the lack ('I have a father') and simulta-neously the beginning emotional investment in her experience of him (and therefore of herself) expressed as 'who acts as if he has no children'. This latter realization points toward what was in retrospect recognizable as a fuller mourning process. From this point of view, rather than a stasis, the aporia outlines the beginning work of mourning, itself always counterbalanced by the pressure to deny the lack of representability (Botella and Botella, 2005).

Notes

1 An aporia is an irresolvable internal contradiction or logical disjunction in a text, argument or theory
2 In fact, trauma can be defined as experience which cannot be represented.
3 In the sense described by Freud (1940 [1938]).
4 I am indebted to Wolfreys for noting the parallel between traumatic experience and aporetic logical structure.
5 A simple example of an aporia is 'Everything I say is a lie'.
6 See Scarfone (2017) for a description of *fantasy* building, as opposed to phantasy uncovering, and the fundamental necessity for engagement with a transferentially invested Other to affect this construction of meaning.
7 For a discussion of attacks on linking and evacuative projective identification as efforts to communicate, see Bergstein (2015).
8 The *addad* are words which carry opposite meanings: for instance, a word which can mean black or white.
9 His derision is obvious when he writes 'When someone suggests to you a solution for escaping an impasse, you can be almost sure that he is ceasing to understand, assuming that he had understood anything up to that point' (p. 32).

10 Her remarkable description is very reminiscent of Botella's (2014) description of a state of *regredient* mental functioning.

References

Bergstein, A. (2015). Attacks on linking or a drive to communicate? Tolerating the paradox. *The Psychoanalytic Quarterly*, 84 (4): 921–942.

Bion, W.R. (1958). On arrogance. *International Journal of Psychoanalysis*, 39: 144–146.

Bion, W.R. (1959). Attacks on linking. In *The Complete Works of W. R. Bion*, Vol. 6. Ed. by C. Mawson (2014). London: Karnac. pp. 138–152.

Bion, W.R. (1976). Four Discussions. In *The Complete Works of W. R. Bion*, Vol. 10. Ed. by C. Mawson (2014). London: Karnac. pp. 51–102.

Bion, W.R. (2013 [1967]). Notes on memory and desire. In *Wilfred Bion: Los Angeles Seminars and Supervision*. Ed. by J. Aguayo and B. Malin. London: Karnac. pp. 136–138.

Botella, C. (2014). On remembering: The notion of memory without recollection. *International Journal of Psychoanalysis*, 95 (5): 911–936.

Botella, C. and Botella, S. (2005). *The Work of Psychic Figurability: Mental States without Representation*. London: Brunner-Routledge.

Brown, L. (2011). *Intersubjective Processes and the Unconscious*. Abingdon: Routledge.

Civitarese, G. (2010). *The Intimate Room*. Abingdon: Routledge.

Civitarese, G. (2015). Transformations in hallucinosis and the receptivity of the analyst. *International Journal of Psychoanalysis*, 96 (4): 1091–1116.

da Rocha Barros, E.M. and da Rocha Barros, E.L. (2011). Reflections on the clinical implications of symbolism. *International Journal of Psychoanalysis*, 92: 879–903.

da Rocha Barros, E.M. (2013). Dreaming and the expressive function of the mind: Transformation from emotion to meaning. Paper given at The Boston Psychoanalytic Society and Institute, December 7.

Derrida, J. (2000). *Demeure: Fiction and Testimony*. Trans. by E. Rottenberg. Stanford, CA: Stanford University Press.

Derrida, J. (2006). *Aporias*. Trans. by T. Dutoit. Stanford, CA: Stanford University Press. (Original work published 1993).

Eaton, J.L. (2011). The obstructive object. In *A Fruitful Harvest: Essays After Bion*. Seattle: Alliance Press. pp. 17–33.

Eshel, O. (2013). Patient-analyst 'withness': On analytic 'presencing', passion, and compassion in states of breakdown, despair, and deadness. *The Psychoanalytic Quarterly*, 82 (4): 925–963.

Ferro, A. (2009). Transformations in dreaming and characters in the psychoanalytic Field. *International Journal of Psychoanalysis*, 90 (2): 209–230.

Ferro, A. (2012). Creativity in the consulting room: Factors of fertility and infertility. *Psychoanalytic Inquiry*, 32 (3): 257–274.

Freud, S. (1900). *The interpretation of dreams*. S.E. 5. London: Hogarth. pp. 339–628.

Freud, S. (1915). *The unconscious*. S.E. 14. London: Hogarth. pp. 159–209.

Freud, S. (1940 [1938]). *Splitting of the ego in the process of defense*. S.E. 23. London: Hogarth. pp. 271–278.

Green, A. (1999). *The Work of the Negative*. London: Free Association Books.

Green, A. (2000). The central phobic position: A new formulation of the free association method. *International Journal of Psychoanalysis*, 81 (3): 429–451.

Grotstein, J. (2007). *A Beam of Intense Darkness: Wilfred Bion's Legacy to Psycho-analysis.* London: Karnac.

Levine, H.B. (2010). 'The consolation which is drawn from truth': The analysis of a patient unable to suffer experience. In *Bion Today.* Ed. by C. Mawson. Abingdon: Routledge. pp. 188–211.

Levine, H.B. (2012). The colourless canvas: Representation, therapeutic action and the creation of mind. *International Journal of Psychoanalysis,* 93: 607–629.

Levine, H.B. (2015). The transformational vision of Antonino Ferro. *Psychoanalytic Inquiry,* 35 (5): 451–464.

Miller, P. (2014). *Driving Soma.* London: Karnac.

Mitrani, J. (2001). *Ordinary People and Extra-Ordinary Protections: A Post-Kleinian Approach to the Treatment of Primitive Mental States.* London: Brunner-Routledge.

Ogden, T.H. (2005). *This Art of Psychoanalysis: Dreaming Undreamt Dreams and Interrupted Cries.* Abingdon: Routledge.

Ogden, T.H. (2008). Bion's 4 principles of mental functioning. *Fort Da,* 14: 11–35.

Plato (1967). *Plato in Twelve Volumes,* Vol. 3. Trans. by W.R.M. Lamb. Cambridge, MA: Harvard University Press.

Roussillon, R. (2011). *Primitive Agony and Symbolization.* London: Karnac.

Scarfone, D. (2014). The unpast, actuality of the unconscious. Monograph for The Actual in Psychoanalysis, 74th Congress of French Speaking Psychoanalysts, Montreal, May 29–June 1.

Scarfone, D. (2017). Fantasy and the process of fantasy-building. Paper presented at the Boston Psychoanalytic Institute and Society, December 2 (Originally published in 2016 as Fantasme et processus de fantasmatisation. *Revue Française de Psychosomatique,* 50: 47–68).

Williams, P. (2007). The body and mind (including of the analyst) in the treatment of a psychotic state: Some reflections: Commentary on a paper by Riccardo Lombardi. *Psychoanalytic Dialogues,* 17 (3): 401–409.

Winnicott, D.W. (1974). Fear of breakdown. *The International Review of Psychanalysis,* 1: 103–107.

Wolfreys, J. (2002). Trauma, testimony, criticism: Witnessing, memory and responsibility. In *Introducing Criticism at the 21st Century.* Ed. by J. Wolfreys. Edinburgh: Edinburgh University Press. pp. 126–148.

Chapter 6

The hallucinated Field

Rodrigo Barahona

Through its original contributions to the exploration of subjectivity and intersubjectivity in psychoanalysis, Bionian Field Theory,[1] has rigorously placed the expansion of subjectivity front and center in clinical practice. While not a Field Theorist himself,[2] Bion's intensely intersubjective perspective on psychoanalytic interaction has helped seed contemporary theorizing on the analytic Field with truly 'wild thoughts'. In this chapter, I will focus upon Bion's (1984b [1965]) theory of transformations, especially transformations in hallucinosis, T(H), and their place in Antonino Ferro's Field Theory. I hope to show how the T(H) concept reflects a state of stasis or contraction in the Field and relates to the formation of what the Barangers (1961–1962) called 'bulwarks' or 'bastions'. These (hopefully) temporary obstructions to analytic process are both necessary and inevitable and have great communicative value. They are central 'knots' in the analytic process that must be untangled as the analysis progresses. Their appearance helps us to notice movements related to the progressive and regressive poles in the analytic Field, states of expansion and contraction that are interconnected with similar states in the subjectivities of the analytic couple. Recognition and working through of these bastions are an important part of what makes the Field concept a useful clinical tool. Awareness of their origins in T(H) offers a valuable vertex to the analyst in regard to the intersubjective flow that takes place in the process.

Like the analytic Field itself, transformations move in both directions, towards expansive and contracting poles. To the extent that T(H) reflect a state of stasis or contraction in the Field, they become a valuable, if not indispensable area of study that can help us understand and make use of moments of seemingly irresolvable impasse, resistance, symptomatic eruption, or negative therapeutic reactions. T(H) are ongoing phenomena in every mind, more usually concealed by other modalities of psychic functioning (Ferro and Civitarese, 2015, p. 145). They provide important points of contact with the psychotic parts of the patient's mind. Their presence may be signaled by the analyst's subjective experience of pragmatic or concrete thinking and boredom, enactments between the analytic pair, or as I will describe in a

DOI: 10.4324/9781003168034-6

clinical example, a frank hallucination had by either member of the couple. These are moments when the Field becomes hallucinated, or in Ferro's terminology, when the Field 'contract(s) the patient's illness' (Ferro, 2015, p. 516; my parentheses).

Transformations

> Saint Paul has described it beautifully: 'Behold I tell you a mystery. We shall not all die, but we shall all be changed'.
>
> (Bion, 1986b [1982])

Introduced by Bion in 1965, *transformations* is a term used to refer to the process a patient's experience undergoes as it changes from one form or state to another. The feature of that experience that remains as an intrinsic component of the patient's inner state, persisting across various representations, is called an *invariant*. The dynamic nature of the representational process is such that the invariant can appear in many manifestations, including the analytic interpretation. Hence, Bion's (1984b [1965]) remark: 'An interpretation is a transformation; to display the invariants, an experience, felt and described in one way, is described in another' (p. 4).

Inhabiting different forms and oscillating between degrees of clarity, these invariances may be grasped intuitively through the analyst's subjective experience. Once they are represented in a form and thus articulated in the analyst's mind, they may be communicated to the patient in a manner that can assist in expanding his subjectivity by transforming and making accessible a previously inaccessible though vital part of his mind.

Field Theory and transformations in the Field

Transformations can be thought of as existing on a spectrum that includes rigid-motion transformations, projective transformations, transformations in hallucinosis, transformations in K and transformations in O (Bion, 1984b [1965]; Civitarese, 2015; Sandler, 2015). Bion writes that 'the term "transformation" may mislead unless the limitations of the implications of "form" are recognized' (1984b [1965], p. 12). In other words, 'something trans-forms itself but something remains the same' (Sandler, 2015, p. 775). That remnant is the invariant, as Bion explains in the opening of *Transformations*:

> Suppose a painter sees a path through a field sown with poppies and paints it: at one end of the chain of events is a field of poppies, at the other a canvas with pigment disposed on its surface. We can recognize that the latter represents the former, so I shall suppose that despite the differences between a field of poppies and a piece of canvas, despite the transformation that the artist has effected in what he saw to make it take

the form of a picture, *something* has remained unaltered and on this *something* recognition depends. The elements that go to make up the unaltered aspect of the transformation I shall call invariants.

(1984b [1965], p. 1)

Here Bion is making an epistemological point: the essence of the poppy field can never be fully captured, or fully rendered by any one representation or transformation of its O. However, its essence – or better put, an essential part – can be represented or alluded to in many different ways, each of which relate to that which is invariant. The same may be said of a patient's separate but similar dreams, where each transforms invariants in the patient's subjectivity, capturing something essential about his psychic functioning, without any of the dreams being able to fully capture its essence.

Not unlike the poppy field, the analytic Field 'is a multi-verse' (Ferro and Civitarese, 2015, p. 73); different characters that are spoken of and so arrive in the Field (a hallucination or the patient's spouse, for example) may refer to the analyst or the patient, to something in the patient's outside life, to a quality of the Field generated together with the patient, to something in the present, past or future, to something conscious or unconscious, etc. (p. 73). For this reason, we can say that the analytic Field is a projection of the conscious and unconscious subjectivities of the pair. Ferro and Civitarese (2015) write:

the space of the analytic Field is unstable/dynamic. It is ever shrinking or expanding. It shrinks when it is invaded by a violent emotion and imposes an absolute view of things; whereas it expands when the play of the characters makes possible multiple points of view on things.

(p. 75)

The analyst's emotional disposition – a feature of his subjectivity – shapes his role as a container to the patient's contained and facilitates transformations of emotion. Ultimately, it is in recognition of the Field's quality as locus and medium of the container–contained dialectic (Ferro, 2009, p. 210) that we say that it is co-constructed. To amplify this quality of the Field, we might also say that it is potentially seen as co-generative and co-inhibitive, as within this dialectic of container–contained are two subjects who alternately embody the poles of *representational imperative* (Levine, 2012) – the inherent, perhaps hard-wired pressure to form representations intrinsic to every mind – and the representational potential of reverie as described in Bion's (1984a [1962]) theory of alpha function and container/contained – the hard-wired disposition in the other to receive signals and create representations from them. These representations will be embedded in a common, socio-semiotic and linguistic code spanning the range from rudimentary visual pictograms (ideograms in Bion's terminology) to more structured, sophisticated, secondary-process and affect-laden narratives.

In the clinical hour, the analyst may intuit the invariances through his use of free-floating attention and by abstaining from memory and desire. The new forms in which invariance may be expressed often reflect the 'selected fact' of the session. Clusters of the patient's associations contain the forms representing the products of these transformations. Vermote tells us that 'the analyst – being immersed in the flux of ever-changing elements – should try to see the invariants in this flux. These invariants in the ever-changing flow of elements point to the psychoanalytic object' (2011, p. 354). For example, the analyst's sense that the recent tension between himself and the patient is slowly being metabolized, and his accompanying relief and trepidation regarding these signs of progress, is confirmed when the patient begins to talk about his hope and anxiety about the recent meetings and easing of tensions between two world leaders. The analyst may not have been consistently conscious of the fact that he was feeling hope and trepidation – the invariants – following a period of protracted tension, but now, with the patient's words, sees them transformed projectively (Bion, 1984b [1965]). He can now find an opening through which to think about his and his patient's concordant feelings and can now consider them analytically worth mentioning: 'It is a relief, but yet, people don't want to let their guard down. After all those years of tension, you never know when all hell will break loose'. Still later, the patient might be ready to hear the analyst say (and the analyst might be ready to hear himself say), 'You know, you and I have been in a bit of a stalemate too, with you being very angry with me and feeling like I won't budge. But today you seem a little readier for us to move on a little and talk about it, though it's still a little scary to totally let your guard down'.

My own manner of approaching analytic work using the Field concept takes seriously Ferro and Civitarese's recommendations that the analyst refrain from 'active monitoring of the analytic conversation' (Ferro and Civitarese, 2015, p. 91). Therefore, I do not enter the session hour with the Field in the front of my mind. Rather, I initiate and go about my work as any other analyst from any other tradition might, with the only aim of maintaining evenly suspended attention as I wait for the patient's words and emotional investments to slowly shape the narrative of what will occur in the session and what will be available for deepening. As a *background* to perception, the Field vertex is always present in my understanding of the different elements that are introduced into the session as potential carriers of emotionally undigested material in search of elaboration and deepening by myself and the patient. This is particularly true when such moments are the result of an underlying state of transformations in hallucinosis, where meaning is seemingly drained from the experience of the couple and, as I will explain below, what is required is an act of dreaming, as opposed to hallucinating, the Field.

Hallucinations and transformations in hallucinosis

I would now like to discuss the concept of hallucination, narrowing on Bion's point of view, in relation to the properly Bionian concept of hallucinosis. This I think is vital if we are to understand the process through which transformations in the form of *hallucinosis* contracts the Field and the subjectivities of both patient and analyst. Others have made the distinction between the two concepts (for example Civitarese, 2015; Guinard, 2015; Hintz, 2015; Meltzer, 2009 [1986]; Sandler, 2015), so here I am merely summarizing some of their thinking. Often, though not always, hallucination forms a part of the state of hallucinosis as both a product of this state and a marker of its underlying existence in the Field.[3] The emergence of a hallucination underlines the presence of a bastion, can call the analyst's attention back to the Field and furnishes an opportunity for the analyst to wake up to the dream of the session. This is especially so when the hallucination can be recognized, through the analyst's alpha functioning, as a new character in the Field (Ferro, 1999 [1992]), allowing for a lower-order or psychotic transformation to provide an opening to a renewed dream-for-two (Cassorla, 2017) of the session.

In short, *hallucinosis* refers to a perceptual *state* of some duration, perhaps better thought of as a process state[4] reflecting an 'inaccessible state of mind' (Bergstein, 2018, p. 202), while *hallucination* refers to an acute perceptual event that is the product of this inaccessible or psychotic state of mind. For Bion, a state of hallucinosis is always present as an underlying condition of the mind, a 'background' (López-Corvo, 2003, p. 137), both normal and pathological (Bion, 1986a [1970]) from which hallucinations may emerge. According to Meltzer (2009 [1986]), the difference between the two lies in the fact that hallucinosis does not involve the perception of *objects* that are not there, but rather of *relationships* that are not there. In line with this, hallucinosis, or transformations in hallucinosis, are not *necessarily* linked to pathology and are 'always present as a medium through which other transformations take place' (Sandler, 2015, p. 1143), including transference and projective identification. Hallucinosis exists *within* a system of meaning (Meltzer, 2009 [1986]), in as much as transference and projective identification interact within the 'membrane' (Sandler, 2015) of hallucinosis where meanings circulate within an impoverished mode of thinking (Meltzer, 2009 [1986]). In other words, the thoughts are there, but the thinking is not.

So, while hallucinosis denotes what Bion (1984b [1965]) would refer to as a *process* of transformation (containing other transformations) the term *hallucination* refers to an evacuative *product* of transformation. The evacuation occurs when the process of transformation of the perception of emotional experience into symbolic form (alpha elements) is impeded by anxiety (Meltzer, 2009 [1986], p. 105). Thus, hallucinations consist of evacuated sense impressions, beta elements that for Bion yield not meaning but only somatic sensations of pleasure and pain.

The meaning that *can* be derived from the hallucination to be put to use by the analyst cannot be grasped 'outside the conditions of hallucinosis' (Bion, 1986a [1970], p. 36) and must therefore be produced through immersion resulting in a transformation from O to K. In other words, the analyst

> must undergo in his own personality the transformation O→K. By eschewing memories, desires, and the operations of memory he can approach the domain of hallucinosis and of the 'acts of faith' by which alone he can become at one with his patients' hallucinations and so effect transformations O→K.
>
> (ibid.)

The contraction and expansion of the analytic Field and of subjectivity

I would now like to turn to clinical material to illustrate the idea put forward in this paper that, in an important sense, the hallucinated Field – in other words, one where hallucinosis is dominant – signals a contraction of the subjectivities of both its inhabitants, and likewise a contraction of the Field's ability to breathe meaning into its objects. The example below, taken from the third and final year of work with Ms. D, a young psychotic woman in an intense, twice a week psychotherapy, demonstrates how a hallucination may perform the function of alerting the analyst to the Field's submerged state in hallucinosis. It emerges at a moment where analyst and patient are 'most vulnerable to the pain of not being able to understand or to give meaning to things' (Civitarese, 2016, p. 42).

Ms. D

Ms. D, a patient with a history of severe psychotic disturbance, had been actively underplaying the discovery of her husband's very large secret credit card debt, drug use and affair with another woman. For the most part, she was pleasant in sessions, had a joking and semi-flirtatious style, and adopted a somewhat overdone, 'don't worry, be happy' demeanor that she proudly claimed was intrinsic to our common Latin American heritage. As a result of my non-casual, analytic focus, she gradually began to regard me as an exception to this cultural feature, and began experiencing the sessions as stressful, often finding herself at a loss as to what to say. Conscious of her fragility and not wanting to increase her anxiety in the session, I accepted her request during this period of our work that we not 'dwell on the negative parts' as she put it, and focus on other, more positive developments that she wanted to discuss. While initially I held in mind the need to address the negative feelings, and the self-defeating ways in which she managed them, over time they receded from importance in my mind. Listening became difficult, and I felt less and less my analytic self. Similarly, my feeling unable to join my patient's casual style had a defensive quality to it, as if I resisted being pulled into something I couldn't bear or understand. My ability to think about the material and my options for intervening felt more and more constricted. Consequently, I found myself offering pragmatic advice on concrete situations that seemed of the upmost importance, and explored themes that only afterwards felt insignificant. While my effort to avoid 'negative topics' was consciously reasoned as a way of keeping the patient's anxiety at a manageable level (the explanation itself a transformation in hallucinosis) I was not aware of the degree to which I was joining my patient in creating bastions in the analytic Field by unconsciously colluding with her.

In one session, however, she batted her eyelids feverishly and, startled, told me that she had just seen a black bird flapping around in front of her, which was now gone. In spite of the fact that the window was closed, she reasoned that the bird must have flown out. When I called her attention to this fact, she said in Spanish, 'Oh, I don't know!', irritated by my questioning her perception. I distinctly remember thinking at that moment how the hallucination of the flapping black bird was facilitated by the impression in her field of vision of her opening and closing eyelids. I *now* regard this half-concretized formulation as an example of how deeply mired I was in a shared state of hallucinosis with my patient, where I viewed the black bird from a concrete physical vertex rather than as an affective hologram. Emerging from this confused and concrete context, the image of the black bird now appearing in my mind as if in a dream, I was able to say, 'un ave de mal agüero', which in English means 'a bad omen bird'. I added that perhaps there was 'bad news' we weren't talking about, and I began to take up some of the inconsistencies of what she had been telling me, and suggested we look at them more deeply. With some anxiety, she began filling me in on the less rosy details of her current situation at home.

Discussion

In retrospect, I was feeling somewhat paralyzed and jarred by the discrepancy between the seriousness of what was happening to Ms. D and the aloofness with which she presented in the session. Unable to process all of this, and affected by her anxiety, my representational capacity was constricted and the container–contained dynamic of the Field shut down. Anxiety increased and Ms. D's ability to connect to her own feelings and therefore to 'think' of what to say became increasingly inhibited. We each lost our sense of ourselves, but hallucinated new ones where she became a positive-minded patient with pragmatic problems to be solved and I, a hopeful and helpful analyst with pragmatic solutions to give. This situation could not last, as it consisted of pseudo-thought, and could be best described as a 'non-dream-for-two' manifesting itself in a transformation in hallucinosis (Cassorla, 2017), which eventually produced a hallucination (the black bird) that evacuated the unthinkable but disturbing elements.

This hallucination, however, *also* offered us an opportunity to re-dream the Field. The ability to think of the bad omen interpretation represented a transformation in *my* mind, though not yet the patient's. It reflected my return to the Field vertex, where I was more attuned to the painful emotional undercurrent of what the patient and I had been avoiding. In other words, back as the possessor of the alpha-functioning for the couple, the patient's hallucination was a curiosity for *me*, and it demanded interpretation of some form in *my* mind. But for the sudden appearance of the bad omen, the patient and I had been, so to speak, living the non-dream (Barahona, 2020) of excitement over her new house, her renewed motivation to get back to work and school, and a re-ignited passion for her husband. The devastating emotional reality of what we had *not* been talking about, but had allowed to take flight out the window, were her feelings of powerlessness and rage over the probable repossession of the house and her husband's affair and worsening addictions, which coincided with my increasing sensation of inhabiting a false self. Re-cast in this way, the black bird helped transform these undercurrents into realities that were more palpable and thinkable in my mind.

This brings us to the transformative nature of the interpretation of a visual hallucination. My intervention did not induce the patient to 'decode' the hallucination, which, after all, is an aborted effort to encode unbearable experience into alpha, which is then evacuated under the pressure of anxiety (see Meltzer, 2009 [1986]). What is never encoded cannot be 'decoded'. It did, however, reflect the fact that I was now back in touch with my own transformational processes and helped produce an idea that, now conscious and shared with Ms. D, became thinkable. The emotions linked to this idea – the *actual* bad news to come – were now susceptible to transformation in Ms. D's mind if handled sensitively in the ensuing dialogue centered around more relevant and tangibly felt material. In short, the interpretation reflects the analyst's regaining access to his intuition and his representational capacity and assists him in guiding his patient back to hers.

In retrospect, a more saturated interpretation could have explicitly conveyed to the patient not only the existence of feelings that were being avoided, but the tendency in the patient to avoid painful emotions, automatic and in the form of evacuation. An example of such a Field-oriented interpretation would have been, 'I think that the magic of a black bird appearing and then flying away through the closed window can tell us what you might want us to do with your very real problems: give them flight and make them disappear'. This might have enabled the patient to notice this tendency in herself and raise it into consciousness by lending it words, words that we could return to in the recursive process of representation and transformation of anxiety. Her field of subjectivity would thus be widened as she experienced and tolerated knowing more about herself and her self-undermining ways of managing her feelings. The interpretation that I did give her, however, allowed us to sufficiently resume our footing in the Field in a way that could be described as waking up from a non-dream-for-two (Cassorla, 2017).

Having gained more traction, I was able to take note in our subsequent sessions of our tendency to 'take flight' from difficult emotions when they reared their heads through the patient's words. Gently bringing them to our attention, I kept in mind my now conscious role as the bearer of bad news bird. Ms. D became more open about feeling angry with me for 'forcing' her to think about her problems. However, I did not notice any defensiveness on my part in the face of her protests, and felt her complaints to come from a place of openness and diminished fear of what her anger might unleash. At the same time, she reported being more direct with her husband, who as a result had begun consulting with a specialist at their bank about consolidating their debts. She also wondered if it would make sense to speak to a divorce lawyer to get a better view of her options. I took both of these developments as signs of Ms. D's growing contact with her emotions and her tolerance for new ideas. Along with greater contact with emotional reality came a clearer appreciation of external reality and a new view of her options. These, in turn, gradually led to a growing sense of herself as someone capable of managing on her own.

However hard-won these advancements, contraction in the Field soon reoccurred, signaling further transformations in hallucinosis and the appearance of new bastions. In the weeks and months that followed, Ms. D at times reverted to a passive stance and avoided speaking of matters pressing in her mind so as to not feel overwhelmed. I noticed myself feeling the growing urge to push her into taking her life into her own hands, while feeling irritated at what I felt was pressure from her to take charge as if she were a helpless little girl. I held these ideas and feelings in mind as I followed her narrative throughout the hours.

Ms. D was concerned about the effects of a hurricane that had recently devastated her home country. She had spent several days trying to get in touch with her mother and father, and only the day before was able to speak with them. She had been stressed and overwhelmed, and had begun hearing the sound of a child crying and of a dog barking outside her house, only to find nothing there when she checked. The appearance of these auditory hallucinations reminded me of feeling overwhelmed with having to take care of a helpless little girl. But, subsumed as I was by the patient's and my own anxiety over the plight of her parents, I failed to recognize the hallucinations as a sign of an underlying state of hallucinosis. Thus, I began talking to her about her own feelings of being like a terrified helpless child or dog, afraid that she will be devastated by the coming storm of all of her problems, and worried that I wouldn't hear this in her nor be able to help her (like her parents who she could not contact).[5] The patient ended this session by talking about her irritation with her father for not having prepared for the hurricane and ensuring *that they would not lose touch*. It was only after the session had ended that I understood that I had *lost touch* with my patient's anxiety by becoming subsumed in a transformation in hallucinosis where I had become excessively concrete in my analytic technique of translating the characters in the Field directly and immediately into internal objects, instead of accompanying my patient in her terror about her parent's whereabouts. In fact, a bastion had been appearing unnoticed for some time prior to this session where I was concretely becoming the lost father who was not receiving my patient's communications. Although I had included this in my interpretation of what I felt was occurring unconsciously in what the patient was saying, the emotional Field of the moment was flooded with anxiety and contracted. Thus, this act of interpreting – as opposed to staying on the surface with the real parents – transformed me into the real parent who had momentarily disappeared and left the patient alone to her anxiety. Had I understood this at the time, I could have put this into words to the patient, and helped to contain and make thinkable her anxiety.

The following session, however, Ms. D began talking about feeling powerless and enraged at her husband who had resumed his massive pot intake. She added that she had an urge to minimize this to me at the moment, but would not, signaling to me that she had regained her ability to use me as a container for her emotions. In the sessions that followed she reported feeling that although difficult, the week had felt 'more in her control'. She had had a long discussion with her husband, who seemed to show interest in making changes in his behavior. She had also decided to give up on what had seemed an unrealistic idea to get accepted into a prestigious university for which she was not qualified, but that she had used as an excuse to not get back into the job market. My sense of these sessions was that Ms. D was able to regain greater contact with reality, and, as with her husband, was experiencing me as making changes in my ability to take in her emotions. Alongside of this came transformations in the way she experienced herself, more capable yet reasonably limited, and therefore less in need of omnipotent defenses to maintain a precarious sense of stability.

At this point in our work, Ms. D was able to take back into herself her feelings of powerlessness and rage, previously projected out into the Field, in the forms of a black bird, a devastating hurricane, the missing parents, the barking dog and the crying child. More capable of tolerating and thinking about her feelings, Ms. D became more secure in her relationship to the world. Shortly after these sessions, and fully installed in her first job in over a decade, Ms. D felt well enough to finish her treatment.

Final thoughts

Bion's model of the personality relies on the theory that elements intrinsic to psychic functioning, in health or pathology, undergo constant states of transformation, in directions that expand or constrict the mind and its ability to think. For Bion, thinking is the ability to make use of experience, always defined by him as emotional experience. When Bion's theory of transformations is placed squarely within a Field model that registers and tracks emotional experience, the analyst's awareness of inaccessible or warded off elements of his own and his patient's subjectivity comes to play an important role in learning about what is happening in the room and moving the analysis forward. Moments of hallucinosis consist of transformations that constrict the analyst's awareness of what is happening and holds the analysis at a standstill. At their worst, transformations in hallucinosis can devolve into disabling psychotic functioning for the patient and threaten to destroy the treatment if not properly tended to by the analyst. Yet, they are also signals and opportunities, as they may be transformed into acute symptoms like a hallucination, retroactively signaling the presence of a hallucinated Field while proactively jolting the analyst awake from hallucinating to dreaming the Field.

Notes

1 More a psychoanalytic tool (Neri, 2013) than a school of thought, 'Field Theory' itself does not refer to a monolithic group and in fact contains various related but divergent strains, each with its own model of mind and therapeutic action. For a comprehensive overview of the different field theories, see Katz (2017).
2 Ferro and Civitarese (2015) note that Bion never used the metaphor of the field to apply to his own work, but suggested Field Theory as an area in need of further development in a letter to Rickman (see Conci, 2011). Bion's own ideas on basic assumptions as unconscious group fantasies, valences and the proto-mental area of the mind all move in this direction (Ferro and Civitarese, 2015, pp. 3–5).
3 It is beyond the scope of this paper to properly delve into the topic, but in this way, the relationship between hallucination and hallucinosis is similar to that made by Cassorla (2017) between chronic and acute enactments.
4 I am loosely adapting this concept from computer science to describe when 'processes' themselves comprise 'states'.
5 Citing Pao (1979), De Masi (2006, p. 119) differentiates auditory hallucinations from visual ones in that the latter appear in the sub-acute phase of psychosis, while the former in the acute phase proper. As this is the case, the patient has access to more ego-functioning (perhaps as a result of an increase in alpha functioning?) and the auditory hallucinations are experienced as ego-dystonic. De Masi suggests that since there is a higher degree of ego functioning, the hallucinations may express conflicts and needs and be therefore useful in understanding the patient and gives an example of directly interpreting an auditory hallucination to a patient, causing them to stop (p. 120). It may be that the fact that the hallucination in these cases is experienced as ego-dystonic engenders curiosity and increases the impetus towards representation in the ego, in the way that anxiety, when not overwhelming, encourages the ego towards symbolization.

References

Barahona, R. (2020) Living the non-dream: An examination of the links between dreaming, enactment, and transformations in hallucinosis. *Psychoanalytic Quarterly*, 89: 689–714.
Baranger, M. and Baranger, W. (1961–1962). La situación analitica como campo dinámico [The analytic situation as a dynamic field]. *Revista Uruguaya de Psicoanálisis*, 4: 3–54.

Bergstein, A. (2018). The psychotic part of the personality: Bion's expeditions into unmapped mental life. *Journal of the American Psychoanalytic Association*, 66: 193–220.

Bion, W.R. (1984a [1962]). *Learning from Experience*. London: Karnac.

Bion, W.R. (1984b [1965]). *Transformations*. London: Karnac.

Bion, W.R. (1986a [1970]). *Attention and Interpretation*. London: Karnac.

Bion, W.R. (1986b [1982]). *The Long Weekend*. London: Free Association Books.

Cassorla, R.M. (2017). Stupidity in the analytic field: Vicissitudes of the detachment process in adolescence. *International Journal of Psychoanalysis*, 98: 371–391.

Civitarese, G. (2015). Transformations in hallucinosis and the receptivity of the analyst. *International Journal of Psychoanalysis*, 96: 1091–1116.

Civitarese, G. (2016). Reverie and the aesthetics of psychoanalysis. In *From Reverie to Interpretation: Transforming Thought into the Action of Psychoanalysis*. Ed. by D. Blue and C. Harrang. London: Karnac. pp. 39–53.

Conci, M. (2011). Bion and his first analyst, John Rickman (1891–1951): A revisitation of their relationship in the light of Rickman's personality and scientific production and of Bion's letters to him (1939–1951). *International Forum of Psychoanalysis*, 20: 68–86.

De Masi, F. (2006) *Vulnerability to Psychosis*. London: Karnac.

Ferro, A. (1999 [1992]). *The Bi-Personal Field: Experiences in Child Analysis*. London and New York: Routledge.

Ferro, A. (2009). Transformations in dreaming and characters in the psychoanalytic field. *International Journal of Psychoanalysis*, 90: 209–230.

Ferro, A. (2015). A response that raises many questions. *Psychoanalytic Inquiry*, 35: 512–525.

Ferro, A. and Civitarese, G. (2015). *The Analytic Field and its Transformations*. London: Karnac.

Guinard, F. (2015). Commentary on 'Transformations in hallucinosis and the receptivity of the analyst' by Civitarese. *International Journal of Psychoanalysis*, 96: 1117–1124.

Hintz, H. (2015). Commentary on 'Transformations in hallucinosis and the receptivity of the analyst' by Civitarese. *International Journal of Psychoanalysis*, 96: 1125–1138.

Katz, M. (2017). *Contemporary Psychoanalytic Field Theory*. Abingdon and New York: Routledge.

Levine, H.B. (2012). The colourless canvas: Representation, therapeutic action and the creation of mind. *International Journal of Psychoanalysis*, 93 (3): 607–629.

López-Corvo, R.E. (2003). *The Dictionary of the Work of W.R. Bion*. London: Karnac.

Meltzer, D. (2009 [1986]). *Studies in Extended Metapsychology: Clinical Applications of Bion's Ideas*. London: Karnac.

Neri, C. (2013). Isabel: Social field, psychological field, and narrative field. *Psychoanalytic Inquiry*, 33: 267–271.

Pao, P.N. (1979) *Schizophrenic Disorders*. New York: International Universities Press.

Sandler, P.C. (2015). Commentary on 'Transformations in hallucinosis and the receptivity of the analyst' by Civitarese. *International Journal of Psychoanalysis*, 96: 1139–1157.

Vermote, R. (2011). Bion's critical approach to psychoanalysis. In *Bion Today*. Ed. by C. Mawson. Abingdon: Routledge. pp. 349–365.

Chapter 7

E pluribus unum

Origins of the analytic Field

Lawrence J. Brown

The central theme in this paper derives from the Latin saying, *e pluribus unum*, the United States' motto that translates as 'out of many, one', which in my view is the essence of what we mean by analytic Field Theory. Briefly put, the analytic Field refers to the emergence of something new arising spontaneously from the unconscious engagement between the patient and analyst. Put another way, Hinshelwood (2018) states that a Field '... means a background out of which something emerges as a figure in the foreground' (p. 1412). It is an emotional experience crafted by barely understood processes from psychic fragments – affects, snippets of memories, phantasies – originating in the analyst's and analysand's representational (and unrepresented) worlds that are combined to create an ambient emotional climate central to the Field that is unique to a moment shared by the analytic dyad, which is subsequently transformed/represented by each member of the analytic pair.

Interest in psychoanalytic Field Theory has burgeoned in the last decade and this paper primarily focuses on three aspects in the development of this concept that I believe have not received adequate attention. The **first** is the early contribution to Field Theory in the work of John Rickman and Wilfred Bion beginning in the early 1940s and through Bion's papers on group phenomena in the early 1950s, eventually leading to the Field theories promulgated by Antonino Ferro and Giuseppe Civitarese. **Second**, I explore in detail the formation of an analytic Field as it appears *in statu nascendi* in the analytic situation and the highly complex processes by which this entity arises in an analysis, relying heavily on the dream theories of Freud and Bion. **Third**, though most papers on analytic Field Theory deal with the analytic couple, the focus in this contribution is on the *dynamics of that Field when three persons are involved*, specifically in analytic supervision. A clinical vignette, which builds on a previous paper of mine (Brown and Miller, 2002), is offered to illustrate the formation of a 'shared illness' in the triadic analytic Field of the analyst, patient and supervisor.

DOI: 10.4324/9781003168034-7

Two books, John Rickman and Wilfred Bion: The early roots of analytic Field Theory

In a peaceful corner of the Mount Auburn Cemetery in Cambridge, Massachusetts, buried among the graves of notable people like R. Buckminster Fuller, Henry Wadsworth Longfellow, Mary Baker Eddy and Edwin Booth (brother of the infamous John Wilkes Booth) lies the unassuming grave of Kurt Lewin. He was educated in Berlin and was a student of Max Wertheimer, one of the founders of Gestalt psychology, a perspective that studied the relation of elements within a structured situation, i.e. that the whole is greater than the sum of its parts. Lewin emigrated to the United States in 1932 and turned his attention to the application of Gestalt theory to understanding the human personality, publishing in 1935 his groundbreaking book *A Dynamic Theory of Personality*, in which he conceived of the personality as developing within a *Field* of multiple vectors – the individual's endowment, the impact of parental input, the cultural zeitgeist – and that one's personality is a unique entity that is greater than the sum of its constituent parts. Interestingly, Lewin's Field Theory began to find its way into the psychoanalytic literature and affected the work of Harry Stack Sullivan (Conci, 2009), Karl Menninger (1937) and Bion and Rickman (1943), and reached as far as Argentina in the early 1940s through the teachings of Pichon Riviere (Brown, 2010, 2011; Etchogoyan, 2005).

A year after the publication of Lewin's well-received book, J.F. Brown (1936) published *Psychology and the Social Order*, about which Menninger (1937) said in the review, 'that all psychoanalysts should read … as an antidote to the extreme individualism' (p. 132) of psychoanalytic practice. While Lewin tended to disparage Freud's work, J.F. Brown emphasized that the theories of Lewin, Freud and Marx were compatible. Pearl King (2003) reports that Rickman read J.F. Brown's book in 1939; thus, Lewin's and Brown's books were slowly introduced to the British Army (Harrison, 2000), which subsequently led to the recommendation by the Directorate of Psychiatry in the War Office to read these two books. Thus, these early notions of a Field Theory seeped into British Army thinking and proved to be a valuable conceptual tool for the Northfield Experiments that Bion and Rickman were to develop.

Bion and his former analyst, John Rickman, began to explore the clinical applications of Field Theory in their early studies of group therapy and together wrote the Wharncliffe Memorandum (Schimmel, personal communication) that proposed treating war neuroses through a form of group treatment; however, several years were to pass before the opportunity came to implement their ideas at the Northfield Army Hospital, where they worked together to develop group-oriented treatments that sought to harness the importance of group process as a therapeutic modality. These early group 'experiments' were of questionable value, but ultimately led to the development of the *therapeutic community* and Bion's con-tinued interest in *therapeutic groups.*[1]

All the influences highlighted thus far seem to have been creatively folded into Bion's theory of group processes (Bion and Rickman, 1961) which skill-fully tied Lewin's concept of the Field with Klein's perspective on unconscious phantasy. In a letter to Rickman (March 7, 1943) (Conci, 2011) regarding what was to be learned from Northfield, Bion commented that 'some very serious work needs to be done *along analytical* and *Field Theory* lines ... But I haven't gotten very far with it' [italics added]. This statement conveys a sense of Bion struggling to bring together Freudian notions with Lewinian Field Theory, an integration that J.F. Brown (1936) had offered earlier. One can speculate that starting analysis with Klein early in 1945 provided him with sufficient first-hand knowledge of unconscious fantasy in order to bring these two intellectual currents (Field Theory and psychoanalysis) together.

Ultimately, Bion learned from his experiences with groups that, given certain situations, a shared phantasy may emerge among group members that is built from the individual psychologies of each person (Bion and Rickman, 1961); however, that phantasy is more than the sum of each patient's contribution. With this recognition, Bion was able to bridge the Freudian/Kleinian concept of unconscious phantasy with Lewin's Field Theory. Put another way, *the emotional Field becomes permeated with the communal unconscious phantasy.* This insight revolutionized our understanding of group processes and set the stage for con-temporary thinking about the analytic Field in individual psychoanalysis.

We may rightly ask, how does this Field and the communal unconscious phan-tasy form? In 'Group methods of treatment' (Bion and Rickman, 1948), Bion spoke of 'shared' or 'pooled' phantasies that arise in the group interactions and also commented on a 'group mentality' or 'group culture' that emerged from 'anonymous [unconscious] contributions' by the group members. Later, in *Experiences in Groups* (Bion and Rickman, 1961), Bion introduced the concept of a *basic assumption* which in essence is a shared unconscious phantasy of the group built from the individual psychologies of each person; however, that phantasy is more than the sum of each individual's psyche. Bion also observes 'how easily and spontaneously it [the group] structures itself' (CW IV, p. 158) around a shared emotional situation and introduces the concept of *valency,* which he defines as 'a readiness to combine all levels that can hardly be called mental at all; that are characterized by behavior in the human being that is more analogous to tropism' (p. 187), to account for this automatic coagulation around a common emotional state to bind the group members. Later, in 'Group dynamics: A re-view' (Bion and Rickman, 1952), he notes that inclusion in a basic assumption is 'instantaneous, inevitable, and instinctive' (p. 236) and depends on each individual's valency, now described as 'a capacity for instantaneous involuntary combination of one indivi-dual with another for sharing and acting on the basic assumption' (p. 237); in essence, birth of the emotional Field from vectors emanating from each group member or, put another way, *e pluribus unum.*

Further steps in the development of the analytic Field

Bion's theories about the formation of the basic assumption in a large group also applied to the emergence of an emotional Field between two people, the analyst and the patient. Willie and Madeleine Baranger (2008 [1961]) are usually credited as offering the first analytic Field Theory by positing the *shared unconscious phantasy of the analytic couple* that 'structures the bi-personal Field of the analytic situation ... [and is] something that is constructed in a couple relationship' (pp. 805–806). It would be inaccurate to attribute their concept of the dynamic Field to Bion's ideas that preceded their classic paper written in Spanish; however, the Barangers and Bion were greatly influenced by, and interpreters of, Lewin's work. It seems likely the Barangers were not familiar with Bion's papers on groups when they authored their classic 1961 paper on the dynamic Field because in 1993, referring to Bion's (1952) work on groups and the existence of unconscious phantasy in the group, they stated that 'This is what we mean by the basic unconscious phantasy in the field of the analytic situation' (p. 17); put another way, that the dyadic analytic Field is a small group.

In summary, the notion of an analytic Field gradually evolved from the Gestalt psychology of Wertheimer and Lewin which was 'imported' to the British Army Office at the outset of the Second World War where it was first applied by Bion and Rickman to develop group-oriented treatment of traumatized soldiers (Northfield Experiments), ultimately giving rise to current thinking on group methods of treatment and the healing powers of a therapeutic community. Following these early innovations, Bion undertook a focused study of therapeutic groups of eight or nine patients and observed that a shared group phantasy, what he was to call a *basic assumption*, readily formed from psychic elements in each group member to create a new entity – the basic assumption phantasy, later to be known as an analytic Field.

Ferro and Civitarese's perspectives on the analytic Field

It is important to note from the outset that Ferro and Civitarese's creative contributions to our study of the analytic Field derive significantly from their creative applications of Bion's work; indeed, they consider their writings 'post-Bionian' in that their books and papers are greatly influenced by Bion's later (post-1962) works, which emphasized alpha function, reverie, dreaming and transformations. Thus, the profundity of Bion's papers from the early 1950s through 1962 dealing with the nature of psychotic thought is given less attention. In addition, most authors who write about the analytic Field typically begin with the Barangers' (2008 [1961]) classic paper and often overlook the early development of the concept in the work of Rickman and Bion; however, in their recent (2015) book, *The Analytic Field and its Transformations*, Civitarese and Ferro alluded to the relevance of Bion's early writings on groups in the development of Field Theory.

> From its inception, the analytic Field was seen as a temporary formation that was unique to the analytic couple, an unrepeatable 'universe' that is born at the beginning of each session, only to be temporarily suspended when each session comes to an end.
>
> (Ferro and Basile, 2009, p. 5)

In addition, this analytic Field is populated by virtual figures which they call *characters* that enter and leave the ongoing dialogue between the patient and analyst. Each of these characters spontaneously entering the Field are essentially *metaphors* which have 'succeeded in expressing all its theoretical and clinical potentialities' (ibid., p. 6), i.e. that are tightly compacted and condensed figures with potential multiple and shifting meanings depending upon the emotional tenor of the Field at the moment. Given the liquidity of the characters entering and leaving the Field, representing a variety of shifting metaphors, the Field itself can have a kaleidoscopic quality in which 'the complex vectorial manifestations ... give rise to turbulence, catastrophic points, and ultimately changes of state' (ibid., p. 7).

Despite the impression of a sort of emotional anarchy in this last quote, Ferro and Civitarese emphasize that the Field is also a container in which the emotional 'violence' (Civitarese, 2013) is contained and transformed through the dreaming function of the analytic pair, Bion and Rickman's (1994 [1992]) notion of 'waking dream thought'. Ferro and Basile (2007) and Civitarese (2013) also envision a *casting agent* under whose direction various 'characters' are chosen to play specific roles in the psychic theater of the intersubjective analytic Field. Of course, these notions of a character and a casting agent are metaphors for capturing the analytic process in the bi-personal Field in which

> The alpha function of the analyst's mind becomes the special locus of the treatment ... [and] one could at this point say, the alpha function of the system made up of the patient-analyst dyad ... To which the two parties contribute to varying degrees.
>
> (Civitarese, 2013, p. 79)

In my view, what is missing from Ferro's and Civitarese's clinically important concepts of characters and the casting agent is that these metaphors do not give sufficient attention to the ways in which the two psyches of patient and analyst interpenetrate with each other to create a new entity composed of elements quarried from each of their psyches. This is considered below in the Discussion section following this clinical illustration.

Clinical illustration: A stagnant Field

Most clinical discussions about the intersubjective analytic Field focus on the relationship between *two people* – the analyst and the patient – and the variety of dynamic interactions which emerge in the analytic process they unconsciously co-author. Their engagement, as we have been discussing, is not simply about these two sovereign individuals, but also involves aspects of each of their internal lives that intertwine through processes of projective and introjective identification and waking dream thought to create the shared unconscious fantasy of the analytic couple. This clinical illustration deals with the complexities when *three personalities* connect with each other in the context of psychoanalytic supervision. These dynamics were explored in a previous paper of mine (Brown and Miller, 2002) in which I state:

> Every supervision, whether of an adult or child psychoanalysis, always involves three people: the patient, the supervisee and the supervisor. Each of these individuals brings his or her psychic makeup to this triadic relationship; thus, there is an engagement of three psyches on conscious and unconscious levels. Furthermore, several dyads also form from these encounters: patient/supervisee, patient/-supervisor, and supervisee/supervisor. Consequently, any supervisory relationship is a complex interplay occurring on dyadic, triadic, conscious, and unconscious levels.

Thus, in parallel with Ogden's (1994) concept of the analytic third, a *supervisory fourth* (Brown and Miller, 2002) unconsciously arises, crafted from the representational and unrepresented worlds of the patient, supervisee and supervisor to form a new entity, the supervisory fourth. Regarding the analytic third, Ogden (1994) comments that

> The analytic third is a creation of the analyst and analysand, and at the same time analyst and analysand are created by the analytic third.
>
> (p. 17)

Similarly, the supervisory fourth is formed from the intersection of the analyst, patient and supervisor, a creation that in turn confers meaning to that triad.

The clinical material I will now present is from the supervision of Dr. F on her first child analytic case. I had previously supervised an adult case of hers as part of her training at another institute. The case, which Dr. F characterized as 'a typical suburban neurotic woman', went well and she now wanted to treat a 'really tough case', especially a child in analysis. Thus, she undertook child analytic training at the Boston Psychoanalytic Institute (BPSI) and requested that I supervise the case. Soon her desire for a 'tough case' was satisfied when Linda, a deeply troubled older adolescent, was referred to Dr. F.

Linda, an attractive and appealing adolescent with significant artistic abilities had recently dropped out of college during her first year, returning home to live with her parents. She grew increasingly depressed, felt like a failure and began to engage in alcohol and drug abuse along with risky sexual behavior.

Her former boyfriend had recently died from a drug overdose and she had regular frightening dreams about him. In the initial consultations, Dr. F found Linda appealing, capable of self-reflection and after several meetings they decided to work together, initially twice weekly which soon moved to three times a week. Linda spoke of her depression over the tragic loss of her boyfriend, but over time gradually began to work through this loss, initially through some risky sexual engagements in order to feel a sense of mastery, and later through a painful mourning process. However, at certain times Linda would limply collapse into a deflated state, seemingly unconscious, as though her life suddenly drained out of her. In supervision, Dr. F and I tried to understand the nature of these anesthetized states, their antecedents and the transference/-countertransference implications: we considered several plausible explanations, but none of these hypotheses proved helpful. However, we were assisted one session by Linda's mentioning a YouTube video in which someone was discussing the notion of a 'core wound' which leaves some people feeling empty and lifeless; somewhat later Linda reported a dream in which she was a toddler who needed help.

Despite these rich associations – the 'core wound' and dream of being a toddler – Dr. F felt that she could not 'locate' Linda in an emotional sense. When I asked Dr. F what she meant by 'locating' the patient she replied that Linda brings up dreams but wants them to mean something else, thereby blocking off the possibility of a deeper understanding of the dream and the patient's sense of being damaged at her core. However, as though demonstrating her sense of being a wounded and helpless toddler, Linda reverted in subsequent sessions to the familiar deflated state that was more apparent earlier in the analysis. Dr. F felt a strong countertransference pull to rescue Linda and in response interpreted, 'There is something about being helpless in bed, paralyzed, comatose, as though you are summoning people to help you'. Linda quickly replied, 'Like my [maternal] aunt', who had been in a coma for many years before dying, which earned her the close and loving care of Linda's mother. This thought reminded Linda that her mother had recently found a diary about the comatose aunt and that her mother suggested that she and Linda read it together. By the end of the session it seemed that Dr. F's interpretation and Linda's meaningful associations to her unconscious aunt were a potential turning point in understanding this symptom and signaled a growing trust in Dr. F (Linda and her mother reading together). However, despite these rich associations, Linda fell back once more into a psychic stupor.

Dr. F began the next week's supervision by wearily saying, 'The treatment feels stagnant. Linda is doing okay, not acting out, having her usual trouble mobilizing herself. Maybe we should consider cutting down our supervision to every other week? I have some other patients that I could use help with'. She also mentioned that Linda's parents were thinking of cutting back treatment for financial reasons. Dr. F, ordinarily an energetic woman, surprised me with her weariness, saying that she had felt this way for some time. I asked why she had not brought this up before and she replied that she didn't want to burden me with this since I recently had a cardiac incident; she was worried about me and thought that I might desire privacy. Her comment made me aware that I hadn't been firing on all cylinders recently and I told Dr. F that I, too, had sensed feeling that the treatment had grown somewhat stagnant (which I attributed to my sluggishness). Our attention turned back to the analysis and Linda's complaints of feeling no energy, that when she talks about her life it feels like it does not belong to her. The session ended with Linda telling her mother that she (Linda) was eating large amounts of chicken flavored potato chips, which her mother said was 'disgusting'. After Dr. F left my office, I had the thought that she and I were trying to 'breathe life into the situation' and that Linda was asking for some life-promoting psychic sustenance.

Thus, the analytic Field shared by Linda, Dr. F and me had unknowingly succumbed to Linda's 'disease' characterized by a sense of weary immobility, our energy sapped and waiting for someone or something to 'breathe life into the session(s)'. If this had been occurring in the usual analytic dyad, one would think of our shared illness as 'an analytic third' in Ogden's (1994) thinking; however, given that there were three members in our Field it seems appropriate to call this contagion 'an analytic fourth' (Brown and Miller, 2002), a presence dominating the ambient emotions in the Field, which had not yet been given representation. Each of us in our own way was experiencing a version of this Field's malady, which according to Ferro and Basile (2009) may be a necessary component of 'curing' the analytic Field: 'Another feature of the field is that it must, however slightly, be infected by the patient's illness, and indeed itself contract that illness' (ibid., p. 7). In the next supervisory meeting, Dr. F said that on reflection 'there was something constipated about the treatment' recently and said she had taken Monday off for an extended weekend to rest up. I also felt more energetic in my recovery which was boosted by remembering the quote from Ferro and Basile that gave me a way of conceptualizing what was going on in the supervision. Linda regularly complained that her 11 am session was too early for her, which prompted Dr. F to say 'I don't think we should give up on that' and was surprised when Linda asked to come to the next session at 11 o'clock, saying 'maybe this week I have more energy'. Shortly afterwards, the weariness reappeared in the session as Linda spoke critically of herself, that she sleeps and watches too much TV while eating strawberries with honey. Dr. F commented that she noticed Linda was waiting for something to be passionate about and that she seems to want her analyst to see her as very ill, which brought the comatose aunt to Linda's mind; then, wondering about her parents, she questioned 'do they really need me to be disabled?'

There seemed to be a sense of opening and increased liveliness in the Field: Dr. F took a long weekend aimed at rejuvenating herself; I was feeling more fully recovered and recollecting the quote from Ferro and Basile enlivened my thinking; also, to our surprise, Linda asked to have an earlier session in order to attend a protest meeting, noting that 'maybe this week I have more energy'. However, the Field started to grow more stagnant again as Linda complained of watching too much TV and eating unhealthy food to which Dr. F interpreted that Linda would like her analyst to see her as very ill. This interpretation appeared to rejuvenate Linda's associative capacity as she linked being 'very ill' with the comatose aunt, which then brought a new thought to mind: that her parents might need her to be disabled. Lastly, and most importantly for this discussion, the Field itself was coming back to life, no longer constipated, as the three of us were partaking of good food, no longer gorging on the 'shit' comfort food.

Discussion: How does the intersubjective analytic Field form?

In the first section of this paper that addressed 'The early roots of analytic Field Theory', we focused on Bion's descriptions of the psychic forces responsible for creating the *basic assumption* which is an unconscious phantasy shared by members of the group. Bion identified several forces at work in the formation of this 'group mentality' or 'group culture' from 'anonymous [unconscious] contributions' by the group members. He observed 'how easily and spontaneously it [the group] structures itself' (CW IV, p.158) by a force he called *valency*, which was a sort of tropism, to account for the pulling together of the group, a process that was 'instantaneous, inevitable, and instinctive' (ibid., p. 216). In addition to these processes at work in group formation, I want to address additional factors involved in the creation of the intersubjective analytic Field, beginning with Freud's (1900) theories of how dreams are formed.

Freud's dream theory addresses the structure of the dream within one person's mind, yet I think the dynamics of that structuring are also applicable to the formation of the intersubjective analytic Field between two or more people. Freud (1905) stated that the building up of the dream was initiated by 'a tissue of thoughts (day residue) … Which has been built up during the day and has not been completely dealt with … [That] joins with an unconscious wish to provide a fulcrum for the dream-work' (pp. 160–161). Dream-work is tasked with creating a disguise for, or 'representing', an unconscious wish so that it may pass through the censor's prohibition and achieve at least partial satisfaction, wish fulfillment, by entry into consciousness. But Freud (1900), always wanting to penetrate a mystery ever further, notes that the dream is not simply a collection of various wishes which are intricately woven together as the dream's 'story', but that each of these wishes is first subjected to a destructive process: 'When the whole mass of these dream-thoughts [unconscious wishes] is brought about under the pressure of dream-work, and its elements are turned about, broken into fragments, and jammed together –

almost like pack-ice' (p. 31). Thus, the dream is created by 'a work of condensation on the large-scale that has been carried out' (p. 279). Put another way, the final dream is like a mosaic that is constructed from unconscious wish-shards, each of which has its own associative clusters and threads, leading to an infinite number of potential dream images created by the dream-work. This process is not unlike a marriage between the genetic (or psychic) bits that combine to create uniquely individual people (or dreams) that had never previously existed. Freud knew as much when he said that even the most thoroughly analyzed dream contained elements that reached into the unknown and eluded analysis.

I believe that the formation of the intersubjective analytic Field follows a similar path to the intrapsychic creation of the dream, but the individual tesserae of the mosaic are not only the fragments of unconscious wishes; instead, the analytic Field is composed of psychic material from analogous regions of the analyst and patient that are brought together through a process akin to condensation. However, in this situation there were three actors – Linda, Dr. F and myself – who composed one triad and three analytic couples (Linda/Dr. F, Linda/me, Dr. F/me), each of whom brought our individual psychic worlds to the supervisory sessions. In this regard, following Bion's theories of groups, at the particular moment under discussion here, our supervisory threesome slowly began to coagulate around the theme of *stagnation* that at first was seen as solely Linda's problem. Dr. F and I in our weekly supervisions discussed Linda's 'pathology' as it manifested in her relationships as well as in the transference/countertransference situation.

Thus, the question may be raised: but what process and through which psychic agency is the shared unconscious phantasy, the intersubjective analytic Field, of the hour organized? Bion observed 'how easily and spontaneously it [the group] structures itself' (CW IV, p. 158). In addition, in the immediacy of the analytic session, affects that arise in the internal worlds of the patient and analysand (and supervisor) are compressed together to create the shared analytic Field (shared unconscious phantasy of the couple/triad or a basic assumption) populated by an infinite number of potential chimeras that are bonded together through condensation; a Field centering around a central affect created from many sources which 'demand representation' (Levine, 2012) by each member of that Field. In our supervisory triad, Linda seeded our intersubjective analytic Field with an affect of lethargic inactivity that slowly seeped into Dr. F's and my psyche, gradually infesting[2] each of us with *our version* of what was emotionally occurring in the Field.

Another way to consider this cumulative structuring of the dream's story (or the triad's intersubjective make-up) is to see its similarity to the play of a child who, from a shelf full of many toys, chooses those that best give voice to the theme he or she is developing. Similarly, particular aspects of internal and unrepresented objects in the analyst's and patient's psyches are identified as best suited to represent the emotional coloring of that Field. And just as

Freud described how unconscious wishes in an individual's dream have been deconstructed, so these inner objects of the analysand and analyst (and supervisee) are subsequently broken apart and then reassembled as the intersubjective analytic Field. I think the central emotional core of the Field effects a magnetic-like pull to pick those broken-apart bits that are best suited to represent that Field, not unlike a painter who chooses a certain color to convey a particular mood. Thus, emotional experiences were evoked in each of us, drawn from our inner objects that were compacted together by the centripetal pull of a central affective experience that was subsequently represented as 'stagnation'.

Conclusion

In this paper, two implicit models have been outlined to account for the origin of the intersubjective analytic Field. In some respects they are complementary, yet there are also important differences.

The first, formulated by Ferro and Civitarese, is that metaphorical 'characters' are formed to represent the emotional Field, a process that is under the guidance of a 'casting agent' which designates the best characters to capture the ambient affects of the Field. Their use of metaphors, characters and casting agents is rich and creatively captures how the Field through its 'stagecraft' gives meaning to the 'violence of emotions' (Civitarese, 2013) that often suffuse the intersubjective analytic Field. In my view, however, they do not offer a metapsychology for how these characters are formed and how the casting agent goes about choosing the best actor to play a part in this stagecraft.

I suggest a second pathway in which the formation of the intersubjective analytic Field is created from the integration of unconscious psychic elements (memories; internal objects; those not yet represented, etc.) that have been harvested from each member of that Field, gathered together to form a new entity (analytic third; supervisory fourth; basic assumption) that is more than the sum of its parts, i.e. 'e pluribus unum, out of many, one'. This approach is modeled on Freud's dream theory and the mechanisms of dream-work he outlines, especially the importance of condensation that coheres these disparate elements together. In the case of the psychoanalytic dyad or triadic situation in supervisions, the gathering together of psychic bits from each participant yields a shared emotional experience like a mosaic arising from this intersection that 'demands representation' (Levine, 2012).

Notes

1   Although much of these early attempts to develop group treatments were of questionable success, Bion implemented a 'Leaderless Group Project' that proved to be very useful in officer selection (Schimmel, personal communication).
2   During the supervisory sessions described here, Linda often used the word 'infesting'.

References

Baranger, M. and Baranger, W. (1993). The mind of the analyst: From listening to interpretation. *International Journal of Psychoanalysis*, 74: 15–24.

Baranger, M. and Baranger, W. (2008 [1961]). The analytic situation is a dynamic Field. *International Journal of Psychoanalysis*, 89: 795–826.

Bion, W. and Rickman, J. (1943). Intra-group tensions in group therapy. *Lancet*, 242: 678–682.

Bion, W. and Rickman, J. (1948). Group methods of treatment. In *Proceedings of the International Congress on Medical Psychotherapy*. Vol. 3: 106–109.

Bion, W. and Rickman, J. (1952). Group dynamics: A re-view. *International Journal of Psychoanalysis*, 33: 235–237.

Bion, W. and Rickman, J. (1961). *Experiences in Groups*. London: Tavistock.

Bion, W. and Rickman, J. (1994 [1992]). *Cogitations* (extended edn). London: Karnac Books.

Brown, J.F. (1936). *Psychology and the Social Order*. London: McGraw-Hill.

Brown, L.J. (2010). Klein, Bion and intersubjectivity: Becoming, transforming and dreaming. *Psychoanalytic Dialogues*, 20: 669–682.

Brown, L.J. (2011). *Intersubjective Processes and the Unconscious: An Integration of Freudian, Kleinian and Bionian Perspectives*. Abingdon: Routledge.

Brown, L.J. and Miller, M. (2002). The triadic intersubjective matrix and supervision: The use of disclosure to work through painful affects. *International Journal of Psychoanalysis*, 93: 53–80.

Civitarese, G. (2013). *The Violence of Emotions: Bion and Post-Bionian Psychoanalysis*. New York: Routledge.

Civitarese, G. and Ferro, A. (2015). *The Analytic Field and its Transformations*. London: Karnac.

Conci, M. (2009). Bion and Sullivan: An enlightening comparison. *International Forum of Psychoanalysis*, 18 (2): 90–99.

Conci, M. (2011). Bion and his 1st analyst, John Rickman (1891–1951): A revisitation of their relationship in the light of Rickman's personality and scientific production and of Bion's letters to him (1939–1951). *International Forum of Psychoanalysis*, 20: 68–86.

Etchogoyan, H. (2005). Melanie Klein in Buenos Aires: Beginnings and developments. *International Journal of Psychoanalysis*, 86: 869–894.

Ferro, A. and Basile, R. (2007). *Avoiding Emotions, Living Emotions*. Abingdon: Routledge.

Ferro, A. and Basile, R. (2009). *The Analytic Field, A Clinical Concept*. London: Karnac.

Freud, S. (1900). *The interpretation of dreams*. S.E. 4–5.

Freud, S. (1905). *Jokes and their relation to the unconscious*. S.E. 8.

Harrison, S. (2000). *Bion, Rickman, Foulkes and the Northfield Experiments*. Abingdon: Jessica Kingsley.

Hinshelwood, R. (2018). John Rickman behind the scenes: The influence of Lewin's Field Theory and practice, countertransference, and W.R. Bion. *International Journal of Psychoanalysis*, 99: 1409–1423.

King, P. (2003). *No Ordinary Psychoanalyst: The Exceptional Contributions of Pope John Rickman*. London: Karnac.

Levine, H. (2012). The colorless canvas: Representation, therapeutic action and the creation of mind. *International Journal of Psychoanalysis*, 93: 607–629.

Lewin, K. (1935). *A Dynamic Theory of Personality.* New York: McGraw-Hill.

Menninger, K. (1937). *Review of Psychology and the Social Order, by J.F. Brown Ph.D.* New York: McGraw-Hill Book Company.

Ogden, T. (1994). The analytic third: Working with intersubjective clinical facts. *International Journal of Psychoanalysis,* 75: 3–19.

Chapter 8

Field Theory and child work

Playing on separate and overlapping Fields

Allen Palmer

> However, other persons always intervene in the patient's narrative and phantasy, or even break into the room in the form of a hallucination.
>
> (Baranger and Baranger, 1961–1962, p. 797)

> The analytic couple is a trio, one of whose members is physically absent and experientially present.
>
> (Baranger and Baranger, 1961–1962, p. 797)

The analytic Field, as described by Baranger and Baranger (1961–1962, 2009), is a dynamic bi-personal configuration, including spatial, temporal and functional elements, resulting in an unconscious 'bi-personal phantasy'. While the Barangers referred to the uniformity of the analytic situation with adult patients, child analytic work differs in many respects. Creating the spatial and functional elements in a child analysis to provide the context for an unfolding 'bi-personal phantasy' is complex. Well-known instances of these differences include: the fact that the arrangement for treatment is made with parents and not the child and that the child patient is oriented to the use of the entire spatial setup, moving beyond the stable constraints of the adult patient reclining on the couch. The child plays, acts, draws, makes sounds, sings, talks, silently mimes, etc. The child is often in motion, moving about the consulting room, commonly acting with and upon the analyst's body and extending the spatial boundaries to include the waiting area, hallway and bathroom.

These multi-varied forms of communication are relatively distinct from the verbal communication in free association and the non-verbal communications of the sessile adult analysand. Action commonly predominates the interaction between child and analyst, resulting in fewer opportunities for immediate reflection and reverie in the analyst, as compared to the adult analyst's frequent opportunity for immediate reflection and reverie. While certain adults communicate in action (verbally or otherwise), the qualities of this communicative mode usually present with greater subtlety when compared to work with children.

DOI: 10.4324/9781003168034-8

Brady (2019, p. 417), in her review of Molinari's (2017) book, noted that Molinari suggests that 'it is action that guides reverie in child analysis', adding 'She [Molinari] is well aware that these distinctions are meaningful but not absolute – the way an adult patient strides or tiptoes to the couch are actions within adult analysis'. Furthermore, another distinguishing feature between adult and child analysis is that adults, usually parents, meet with the analyst on a regular basis and accompany their child to sessions, interacting, however briefly, with the analyst at the start and the end of the sessions (Molinari, 2013a), and communicating as well via written, voice and electronic communications.

Nonetheless, in child treatment, the parents' investment in the treatment, the regularity of sessions and the overall spatial elements of the analyst's setting, i.e. the consulting room and auxiliary spaces, provide sufficient contextual components to enable the development of a bi-personal Field, a shared unconscious fantasy and opportunities for narrative expansion, working through and transformations. While the treatment structure provides the context for the clinical encounter, *the Field is a conceptual guiding perspective in the mind of the analyst*. Structural components alone do not constitute the Field. Rather the analyst's perspective is on the here-and-now encounter and the receptivity to the mobilization of unconscious dynamics and co-constructed fantasies in the interpersonal relationship.

The analyst's pre-session thoughts of current-day external events, developmental history, past conflicts, transgenerational influences, family group dynamics, and his or her own personal associations, etc. are considered 'upstream', i.e. antecedent to the analytic encounter (Levine, 2019, personal communication). These may form the background of what facilitates the shaping and elaboration of the unconscious shared fantasy of the Field, but should be seen as the kinds of memories and desires that Bion would have us eschew, because they are potentially obstructive to what will be emergent experiences in the here-and-now. In contrast, similar topics that may occur to the analyst within the session, however, are seen as products of the Field.

The Field-oriented analyst is receptive to the notion of 'illness in the Field', whereby disruptive emotions, or beta elements as per Bion's ideas of the communicative dimension of projective identification, will seek expression, entering and suffusing the Field. This development is potentially accessible for the analyst to grasp, metabolize and interpret to the patient, thereby expanding the patient's capacity for processing powerful proto-emotions in expanded narrative fashion and widening the patient's capacity for representation and thinking. Conceptualized from a post-Bionian perspective, whether considering an adult or child analysis, the Field is the context for the patient's 'waking dream thoughts', the analyst's reveries and the metabolization of proto-emotions, emotions and sensations. The analyst's task is the deconstruction, reformulation and elaboration of waking dream thoughts and the facilitation of the development in the child of 'tools for feeling, dreaming, and thinking' thoughts and metabolizing emotions (Ferro, 2018, p. 115). This is a joint project and, as such, is an evolving, intersubjective co-construction carried out by both analyst and patient. Similarly, Ogden speaks of the analytic task as dreaming the session and dreaming what had been unable to be dreamt by patient and/or patient and analyst before (2005, 2008).

In years past, it was not uncommon for the child analyst to adopt a model of minimal contact with the parents and to assign parent guidance work to another clinician (Isaacs Elmhirst, 1988). Melanie Klein had minimal contact with parents while conducting child analysis, prioritizing the analysis of anxieties associated with unconscious conflicts and internal object relations over environmental influences. When Kleinian adherents conducting child analysis met with parents, contact was limited to a few meetings per year and simultaneous conjoint treatment with another clinician was recommended for them. In contrast, Anna Freud tended to include parents in the analytic endeavor and gave emphasis to external influences in addition to intrapsychic factors.

In the US, the trend has been for child analysts to follow this orientation, by working collaterally with parents and placing a high priority on forming a therapeutic alliance with them. The result is a treatment orientation that frames the analyst's task with parents as facilitating their capacities to foster their child's development. This perspective prioritizes external reality and educational efforts supporting developmental progression and is informed by the analyst's grasp of the child's intra- and inter-psychic conflicts and family dynamics, as well as his or her understanding as to what constitutes developmental progression.

Regarding parent work, Field Theory offers the child analyst a unique perspective that departs from the reality and developmentally oriented perspectives of traditional parent guidance work. The emphasis is on accessing unconscious trends as they emerge in the moment-to-moment encounter with the parents and the analyst's participation in its co-construction. Pressures for reality-, educational- or developmentally oriented interventions are more easily understood as pressures for action that eschew deeper understandings and signs of enactment in the dynamic encounter between parents and analyst. Such pressures may come from parents or other caretakers, such as teachers or pediatricians, or from the analyst's own theoretical orientation and/or anxieties.

The child analyst may use Field Theory to understand the parents' communications about current concerns, developmental events or other matters as reflecting their experience of the here-and-now encounter with the analyst. These communications can create an unconscious interplay between analyst and parents, thereby potentially helping the parents to metabolize powerful emotions so as to widen their tolerance and receptivity and their understanding of their child. While there exists no contract to work with the parents on their personal issues, opportunities exist to work with these very same issues as displacements when the analyst reflects on characters in the parent/child analyst Field and offers unsaturated interpretations and monitors the sequela of these interventions.

From a Field perspective, the analyst can consider the parents' primary focus on their child as a central character in the Field. One might expect parents to introduce other persons in the child's life, such as siblings, friends, teachers, pediatricians, grandparents, medications, alternative therapies, etc., but when they do so, the analyst can also view these as characters in the Field. Rather than the emphasis being on the 'reality' of the persons or situations mentioned or on influential historical experiences, it is on the moment-to-moment emotional encounter, containing nascent representations of unmetabolized emotions and unthought thoughts offering a window into the unconscious processes unfolding between parents and analyst. The analyst immerses him or herself in the parents' concerns, tuning into the emotional tenor of the unfolding story and to his or her own feelings, reflections and reveries. This listening stance allows the analyst to participate in the shaping of the evolving narrative in the bi-personal Field between analyst and parents.

The following case illustrates the complexity of working simultaneously with the child in analysis and collaterally with parents. Furthermore, the case illustrates the creation of a parent/analyst Field and child/analyst Field and how developments in each Field overlap and interpenetrate one another.

> A 5-year-old boy named Spencer was brought to treatment by his mother for temper tantrums, anxiety and enuresis. He was the younger of two children with a brother two years his senior. The parents were recently divorced, and their current interactions were tension-filled bitter disputes around finances, visitation and conflicting views of their child's psychological and medical concerns. The parents requested individual interviews and were seen separately. The analyst first met with Spencer's mother and heard her fears about Spencer's emotional state and reaction to what she described as Father's hostile, emotionally abusive stance toward her and his excessively controlling and similarly emotionally abusive stance toward their children. Examples cited included Father's rigid adherence to schedules, vague indicators of physical contact with Spencer at night, and Father's blocking the children from contacting Mother by phone when ill. She saw her son as fearful of Father, complying with his wishes and suppressing his emotions until he returned to her home, whereupon he disobeyed her and cried inconsolably. Mother sat on the edge of her seat with papers spilling from her lap as she shared this, tearfully distressed and appealing for help.
>
> The analyst felt sympathetic to Mother's concerns and initially drawn into and appalled by the turbulence of emotions and threats she described. The threats felt palpable to the analyst, reflecting the dangers Mother felt for her son and her self. Drawn into a vortex of Mother's distress, the analyst envisioned the father as a monster wreaking havoc in their midst. Initially, the analyst pictured Spencer and Mother as helpless victims and Spencer being unable to manage powerful emotions.

Reflecting further on the initial meeting the analyst toggled back and forth between a reality vertex and a Field Theory vertex. Was there actual emotional abuse occurring and/or was this the unfolding story of a parent contending with overpowering and unmetabolized emotions in herself and in her experience of her child? The former might require interventions by third parties serving containment and the latter a deeper immersion and facilitation of an evolving narrative. To what extent was the fear of the condemning authority who would separate her from her child a projection in anticipation of telling her story to the analyst? And to what extent did the analyst's emotional resonance with the Mother's opening narrative reflect his own anxieties in the face of the powerful forces at play?

The analyst met with Father subsequently and was curious and apprehensive prior to the encounter. The analyst was cognizant of the influence Mother had on him in shaping his anticipations. Who would the analyst meet – the 'monster' from the Mother/analyst Field or someone else? Father, in the initial meeting, calmly and with an air of reasonableness stated he did not understand the purpose of the consultation. He saw Spencer as 'normal' and negated Mother's 'overblown' concerns. While admitting he did not know much about normal development, he saw his son as a healthy boy with typical interests in block building, puzzles, playing with balls and having a typical conflicted sibling relationship with his brother. Furthermore, he felt it important to minimize Mother's influence on their son, seeing his son as a 'people pleaser' and vulnerable to Mother's negative pressures. He saw Mother as being unable to separate from their children during visitation hand-offs, citing Mother's emphasis on how much she and they will miss one another, provoking the children to tears and angry refusals to leave her and go with Father. Father emphasized how imperative it was for him to abruptly end these episodes and hasten the hand-offs.

While Father saw no purpose in meeting with the analyst, he used the opportunity to share his story and perceptions of his son and ex-wife. The analyst felt the Father's skepticism of any necessity for the analyst's involvement. Yet, the analyst also felt an appeal from the Father to view Spencer's mother as unstable and threatening. Here again, the analyst toggled between the vertices of external reality and a Field Theory perspective. What was beginning to be co-constructed in the opening session between Father and analyst? Who was Mother in Father's inner experience – was she a mother unable to separate from her children and unable to foster the children's autonomy and foster a constructive relationship with their father and/or was she dangerously holding on to her children and shaping their perceptions to match her own? The analyst perceived Father as asking him to join forces against Mother as a dangerous influence and to see Father as a steady and collected presence, thereby protecting his sons from actual threats. The analyst thought this appeal might reflect Father's antipathy toward his sons' dependent longings, a negative reaction to Mother's pressures for contact with her sons, and a reaction to Mother's hostility toward him, while also being a response to the analyst's presence and offer of help.

The analyst experienced the powerful emotions in both stories, but ultimately felt that sorting out the accuracy of each parent's external reality was not productive. Both Mother and Father cared deeply about their son's well-being. The question of abuse appeared unlikely. Most important was the analyst's awareness of the dangerous emotional forces in the here-and-now, i.e. how each parent viewed the other as dangerous.

Within each Field a monster came to life in the imagination of the analyst – a Minotaur and a Medusa. While each story sought to influence the analyst toward remedies of riddance or, at the least, containment, the analyst considered the third option of transformation. Using Field Theory facilitated the analyst's movement away from action in external reality (which may have been necessary in circumstances of clear signs of abuse) and permitted the analyst to focus on the transformative possibilities in each of the parent's narratives. The analyst wondered what his first encounter with Spencer would be like. Would the dual parental narratives of helplessness before dangerous aggression be part of the co-created narrative in the bi-personal Field between analyst and Spencer? How was Spencer contending with the powerful emotions and perceptions of both parents and what would emerge in the clinical encounter and the unconscious dialogue between him and the analyst?

Ultimately, both parents were supportive of the child's analysis: for Mother's part, she felt the treatment recommendation validated her concerns about Spencer, and for Father's part, he felt he had no choice but to go along with the recommendations, not wanting to be perceived as obstructionist. As the analysis proceeded, both recognized Spencer's intense engagement in the analytic relationship and supported his use of the process to address his own turbulent, unmanageable feelings. Father gradually saw great benefit in giving his son an opportunity to express his feelings.

Spencer presented as a lively, stout boy with an interest in sword fights and battles. In repetitive fashion, he created barriers and enclaves with office furniture and armed himself and analyst with guns, swords and bombs. The analyst added toy cell phones to the mix, which Spencer readily accepted and used. While this was a spontaneous offering, it reflected the analyst's desire to have a means of verbal communication, a channel for commentary and interpretation within the play.

In the battles that ensued, Spencer would jump out of his redoubt, narrowly defeat and kill the analyst only to revive the analyst and begin again. In dreamlike absorption, Spencer was intensely engaged, acquiring ever more powerful weapons, e.g. 'mega-electric shock' bombs and 'mega-earthquakes'.

The analyst 'felt' the floor quake beneath him and, at times, worried if he would be injured in one of the vigorous sword battles.

Therapeutically, the analyst felt helpless, endlessly defeated. The analyst attempted to manage his sense of futility by clever attacks of his own and comments regarding Spencer's urgent necessity for omnipotent control in order to avoid feeling helpless against dangerous forces. Spencer ignored the remarks and continued in his repetitive play. The analyst came to recognize his own initial efforts as counter-transference enactments, trying to contain the powerful forces at hand. This effort paralleled Spencer's own directives to have the analyst place him (Spencer), 'the bad guy', in jail and stand guard. Spencer would then demonstrate the futility of such efforts, by breaking out and resuming his mega-attacks. At times, Spencer would use his cell phone to call the analyst to purchase greater quantities of ever more powerful weaponry. At other times, he called the 'bad guy police' (another role assigned to the analyst) to capture and jail the analyst-as-foe. In this context, the analyst noted how scared Spencer was of the analyst, 'the bad guy', and how Spencer needed to turn the tables on him; in the face of such danger it was necessary to feel strong and protected from harm.

In retrospect, the 'monsters' within the parents' narratives as well as the powerful emotions within Spencer had come to life in the play and forcefully asserted their place in the child/analyst Field. The analyst experienced the powerful emotions from the overlapping Fields and struggled with vulnerability and impotent helplessness. The analyst experienced within the three intersecting Fields relentlessly powerful forces that could not be contained, civilized or destroyed. From the Field Theory perspective, the shared fantasy had emerged: there seemed to be a persistent choreography repeated in any number of manifestations within the various Fields of unmanageable, violent and destructive forces that could neither be safely contained nor transformed into something more useful and adaptive. This 'casting' also applied to a traditional formulation of the analyst's counter-transference, i.e. feelings of powerlessness in the face of the rage within Spencer and in the Field.

The analyst thought of Spencer as struggling with his own massive destructive forces and tried to help him find creative ways to represent this within the play and the dyadic encounter. The analyst thought of how Spencer had been and continued to be witness to terrible battles, of how Spencer's internal representations of his parents were of each distrusting the other and, on some level, of being scared of one another, and of how Spencer was trying to achieve protection against the destructive forces created by his parents. Furthermore, the analyst thought that Spencer was reliving in the analysis his internal experience of being helpless in the face of overwhelming external and internal destructive forces and projecting this state onto the analyst to help him contain, bear, understand and transform the powerful destructive feelings gripping him.

Notably, his introduction in the play of 'mega-electric shock' and 'mega-earthquakes' and their destructive powers was a creative representation, conveying his complex emotional state. His construction of barriers to create a safe enclave appeared to represent his wish for safety from both destructive forces and possibly from threats of engulfment. Conceptualized through a Field Theory perspective, these representations were characters in the Field, opening up a pathway to first showing and then thinking previously unbearable, complex emotions. Given the immediacy of the evolving co-construction of the narrative, the analyst focused his remarks on the actions and feelings of the play, eschewing interpretations referencing Spencer's external life circumstances and past experiences. As Molinari indicated (2017, p. 11), 'thinking could take place only by allowing the child to continue the process through a figurative representation'.

The analyst's additional thoughts included considering the play as a representation of a boy in the throes of a developmentally normal Oedipal conflict, struggling to destroy and revive the beloved father rival. However, on further reflection, the analyst recognized that viewing Spencer's play as representing a usual developmental struggle risked minimizing this boy's struggles and that association to normal developmental issues was informed by the Father's stance ascendant in the analyst's mind, a stance of downplaying Spencer's emotions. Perhaps the analyst's reaching for a familiar conceptual formula of normalcy reflected his efforts to manage his own turbulent feelings and counter-transference.

Further associations emerged to thoughts of how Mother characterized her ex-husband as an extremely clever manipulator, always seeking control and advantage. Was this, too, a residue from the parent Field with Mother's stance prominent in the analyst's mind? This seemed to be an entry point into understanding the unconscious aspects of the bi-personal Field with Spencer. Was Spencer identified with Father and the analyst with Mother or its reverse, where Spencer was enacting an identification with the helplessly controlled mother and the analyst was the threatening father who needed containment in jail? Or was it Mother whom he needed to contain, given the intensity of her attachment needs and her presumption that she truly knew his inner emotional state? With these cumulative and confusingly interlocking thoughts in mind, the analyst interpreted to Spencer that he was attempting to actualize a wish to be omnipotent via his action, by rendering the analyst weak, helpless and absent of any control. Spencer listened and continued his play as before. Asked if he heard what was said, he replied, 'Oh yes, I heard you, but I'm not going to listen'. It was uncertain if the comment led to an expansion of understanding.

The analyst's desire to be listened to once again reflected the analyst's wish to contain his counter-transference confusion and to persuade

Spencer to move forward with the analyst's understandings, which Spencer rebuffed. In retrospect, this might be considered an ill-timed interpretation serving to benefit the analyst's effort at addressing his counter-transference. Yet, the analyst's position of trying to persuade by offering a saturated interpretation may have represented the pervasive dynamic in the overlapping Fields where persuasion and attempts at coercion substituted for understanding. Father wanted his son to be autonomous, self-contained and free of any dependency needs, whereas Mother wanted her son to be able to remain closely attached, express his feelings without limitations and not morph into a junior version of his father. Each parent was invested in persuading Spencer to adopt his or her viewpoint of the other parent. Rage and intolerable helplessness pervaded the overlapping Fields.

In rare responses to interpretive remarks, Spencer would briefly leave the displacement of the play and comment on his home life, saying that his parents were having 'revenge' fights, that he enjoyed time with both of them and that he saw his father having the most power, his mother half as much, his brother at a 10% level of power and himself at a 5% level. Such quantification led the analyst to associate to the parents' report of Spencer becoming enamored of arithmetic and video games, where power, health and destructiveness were quantified and death and revival were played out repetitively.

The form of Spencer's play evolved as he began to play competitive board games, meticulously learning the rules and quantifying wins and losses. His powerful emotions found a new form of expression in latency-like games. He alternated between playing 'by the rules, fair and square' and playing with cunning stealth. At times, Spencer abandoned all semblance of order, imperiously changing rules at whim, racking up victory after victory. The analyst no longer felt an urgency to interpret Spencer's underlying feelings motivating his actions and, instead, participated in the play with spontaneity and curiosity. At one point, with a wry smile, Spencer announced his intention to spy, explicitly asking the analyst to ignore what he was doing. There was a light-hearted mutual understanding that the analyst would both see and not see what was going on. The analyst felt amused by these playful breaches of the rules and speculated to himself whether this development in the play represented a novel tertiary position, a position beyond competing in a rigid rule-bound contained manner and competing in a state of manic-like exuberance and anger. Could this be the beginning of a transformation in play?

In working with the parents, it became clear that Father reacted to Mother's displays of emotion and general disorganization by intensifying efforts at establishing order and control. Mother, in turn, reacted to Father's strict limitations on her contact with the children during the children's time with him by becoming frantic and disorganized. Each activated the other and each hoped to convince the analyst of the correctness of their perceptions and suspicions.

Mother, for her part, experienced the analyst as an ally, helping her widen her repertoire of ways to help her son talk about his feelings and thoughts. In particular, she asked how she could help her sons when they were barred from communicating with her. When the analyst asked about her own experiences with separations, she burst into tears and recalled painful separations from her parents who devalued her distress about their lengthy absences from her. She remembered their ineffectual offers of toys as substitutes for their presence. The analyst thought of the 'monster' again, but now as an embodied representation of parents who absented themselves from a desperate child, temporarily refusing the child's pleas to remain together. Mother quickly recognized how she had ascribed her own feelings of loneliness and despair onto Spencer and his brother and, for the first time, entertained the possibility that they might be doing well in their father's care. The seeds of transformation were taking root.

Father held to his view of his ex-wife as a pathological influence and cited instances of Mother complicating transitions by clinging to her children during drop-offs. Over time, he spoke with greater spontaneity about how he himself felt out of control in her presence and how this triggered a peremptory need to establish greater order and limits. Father found the analyst to be understanding of his concerns about his ex-wife and helpful in providing a better understanding of his relationship with his son, yet continued to appeal to the analyst to confront Mother's distortions and stop her from pressuring their children to adopt her point of view about him.

Analyst and parents form their own Field, communicating on an unconscious register and shaping an unconscious fantasy. The analyst's associations to his or her analytic work with the child may inform the here-and-now unconscious developments in the Field with the parents. The same can be said for the analyst's recall of the child's and family members' past history or the analyst's personal associations. In parallel fashion, the analyst remembering an emotionally charged interaction with the parents or the parents' reported or demonstrated feelings toward their child informs the analyst about the here-and-now Field with the child. Not uncommonly, unconscious conflicts in parents shape the counter-transference of the analyst toward the parents and act as a powerful 'upstream' vector, influencing the analyst's waking dream process within the bi-personal Field with the child analysand. There is an inevitability of such external vectors entering into the two separate Fields, given the overlapping nature and semi-permeability of the Fields.

While a shared unconscious fantasy can emerge in the parents/analyst Field, such a constellation is invariably beyond the scope of the analyst's role to analyze, since no such agreement has been made between the analyst and the parents. The parents' influence on the bi-personal Field may serve as a positive, background presence, girding the infrastructure of the treatment itself. In the case of Spencer, while the parents were not generally receptive to addressing their individual issues in depth, the child had no doubt of his parents' support of his treatment. A concrete example of this was when he would ask whichever parent was present to negotiate substitute appointments for cancelled sessions and would witness their earnest efforts to do so. Thus, the idea of a supporting, benevolent background presence was in both the patient's and analyst's mind throughout. While there was no obvious representation of this in any specific character in the Field, one wonders if Spencer's sense of safety, in spite of all the destructive forces unleashed, was an unstated entity in its own right. This may be likened to Bleger's ideas on the 'non-ego' aspects of the background, i.e. '"the constants", within whose limits processes occur' (1967, p. 518), forming the frame for the 'organized ego' to develop (p. 513).

Ferro, in presenting a case of working with parents concerned about their son's difficulties with defecating, spoke of imagery emerging into a meaningful narrative that provided insight into the group functioning 'as a single mind' (1999, p. 153). A shared unconscious fantasy of the family group was conceptualized as a unitary 'mind'. Molinari (2013b) extended the family unitary 'mind' concept when she referred to the intersubjective communications between analyst, parents and child, noting the creation of a 'group Field'. The group Field concept encompasses parental and transgenerational influences on the child and, by implication, on the analyst.

Molinari speaks of unconscious developments within the dyadic Field often representing a precipitate of not only the two minds in communication, but also of the Field of the group, which would include parents', and perhaps others', unconscious issues. (Molinari, 2013b). This, of course, would be true for adults too, where the semi-permeability of the Field offers the patient a multitude of entry points for past relationships and influences. According to Badoni the child analyst has the dual tasks of

'taking in' the parents–child relationship he/she tries to help the parents to free the child from their own projections, and by acknowledging the child's perceptions and emotions, the analyst will help the child to define his/her own identity.

(Badoni, 2002, p. 1113)

Molinari (2013b) has conceptualized the Field broadly as an oscillation between a bi-personal Field and a group Field, with the latter including the child, the analyst and the parents. Of note, Molinari (2013b) has cited a case in which a child patient's play and drawings enabled an exploration of the unconscious fantasy in the bi-personal Field of child and analyst and that of the extended, family group Field, including the unconscious relationship between the analyst and the parents:

Elisa's game contained traces of one of my countertransferential senti-
ments toward her father and led me to hypothesize that the drawings, like
the game, could also be considered a tool with which to map the emotions present in an analytic Field that extended beyond the analyst–child
couple. The drawings then were utilized as a probe with which to explore
the universe of emotions that gathered in the Field, rather than being
used in an explanatory sense [with the child and with the parents].

(2013b, p. 308)

Strictly speaking, the Field with the parents does not fall within the usual para-
meters that define a Field with adult analysands. As noted earlier, there is no
contract for an exploration of their inner worlds or for the processing of their
waking dream thoughts. The temporal and spatial aspects of meetings with parents differ radically from the usual analytic arrangement with analysands. The
contract with parents is to help their child overcome their pain, suffering and
obstacles to progressive development. Within this unique context, dynamic factors get mobilized in the relationship between the child analyst and parents and
within the entire family unit (Molinari, 2013b). Given these goals and limitations,
from a Bionian perspective, one can conceptualize the analyst's 'parent guidance'
task as facilitating the development of a flexible container to help parents contain
and metabolize (alphabetize) the proto-emotions of their suffering child and,
perhaps in a more limited way, for themselves. The analyst facilitates the parents'
expansion of the container, their ability to receive their child's projective identifications or beta elements, their ability to metabolize these elements and then their
ability to return them in a more usable form to their child. By adopting the Field
perspective as it relates to work with the parents, the analyst seeks such transformations directly in the here-and-now encounters with the parents. Thus, parents
are helped to promote alpha functioning and the development of new tools to
dream and narrate unmetabolized proto-emotions, emotions and sensations in
the child via their own transformations achieved through their work with the
analyst.

As Badoni points out, while the treatment contract may be to alleviate the
child's symptoms, the parents can be invested in maintaining the family homeostasis and keeping the transgenerational issues unexamined and unthought, i.e.
'curing without curing' (2002, p. 1113). Such resistances can create an unconscious vertex within the parent/analyst Field based on counter-transference reactions to the parents. Negative counter-transference reactions in the analyst may
result in a downgrading of efforts at thoughtful exploration with parents and
result in counter-transference enactments in the analytic work with the child. Two
possible scenarios may ensue: first, the analyst may introduce or amplify themes
of hostility and opposition to the parents within their work with the child or,
second, the analyst may avoid recognizing his or her own reactions and may
comply with the conscious or unconscious parental influence, bringing such
influences to bear in the Field with the child.

Furthermore, the analyst may rationalize their actions as an effort to maintain an alliance with the parents in order to safeguard the analysis with the child or as a reasonable pathway to facilitating the child's development in the child's external world. More subtle reactions include avoidance of the parents' aggression, which could be manifested as the parent's threat to terminate the treatment. The intrapsychic presence within the analyst of the parents' conscious and unconscious agendas can make its way into the psychoanalytic Field via the analyst's counter-transference and via the analyst's departures from Bion's recommendations of entering into the treatment session with no memory, desire or knowledge. There exists a semi-permeable boundary into the Field, and, in this case, the conscious and unconscious parental directives enter the Field consciously and unconsciously via the analyst.

As Ferro (2018) points out, one could approach a child's conversation about a person in his or her life from various vertices that include: a reflection on external reality and the actualities of persons in their lives, a reflection of self and object relations or a reflection on the child's experience of the therapist/analyst and the moment-to-moment developments of the Field. From a post-Bionian Field Theory perspective, the child's reference to parents during their analysis can be viewed as characters in the Field, as well as the child's commentary on his or her experience of what is being dreamed together with the analyst. In the example cited above, Spencer's direct comments about his parents' 'revenge' battles and his power rankings of family members could be viewed either as his perceptions of external reality or as his internal self and object representations, but from the Field perspective, such references were the introductions of characters to the Field, reflecting further elaboration of his emotional experience of the moment-to-moment bi-personal dynamic.

In the formulation of a dynamic bi-personal Field in the analyses of adults, the Barangers introduced the idea of 'a third'. The third was considered as the entry of archaic objects within the dyad emanating primarily from the adult patient, but not exclusive of contributions from the analyst's internal objects. Via projective and introjective processes, the third crystallizes as a created unconscious fantasy between patient and analyst (Baranger and Baranger, 1961 1962; Ogden, 2005, 2008). In considering the conduct of a child analysis where there is intermittent, yet ongoing, contact with the child's parents, conceptualizing 'a third' takes on added complexity. In this instance, the third is created by the child projecting aspects of archaic objects and current day external object relations with parents and by the analyst's openness to receiving and, to an extent, identifying with these elements. Within the context of the dyadic analytic relationship, the child's waking dream thoughts are available for deconstruction, elaboration and interpretation. This process then facilitates narrative expansion in whatever form is in keeping with the child's development, be it verbal narratives, play or drawings. In the separate Field formed in working directly with parents, the child analyst is available to introject and identify with projected aspects from the parents and can unconsciously import these constellations into the bi-personal Field with the child patient. It would seem likely that the work in the parent Field creates a strong valence in the associative possibilities for the child analyst in his or her work in the child Field. This might be especially so if the analyst develops a strong counter-transference position to the parents. In this sense, in child analysis overlapping Fields may exist and the structure facilitating the creation of the Field has a semi-permeable membrane.

Working with parents when conducting a child analysis presents the unique complexity of creating an alliance with parents and mobilizing the parents' conscious and unconscious dynamics and influences, while simultaneously developing a bi-personal analytic relationship with the child. It is somewhat inevitable that a child analyst will be influenced by the parents' agenda beyond the usual therapeutic aims, as the Field is gradually co-constructed. Conceptualized within Field Theory, complex counter-transference amalgams mobilized in the parent/analyst Field can cross the semi-permeable boundary into the analytic Field with the child, contributing to the unconscious fantasy of the bi-personal Field with the child. The analyst's reactions to parents can include unconscious identification or counter-identifications with the parents' conscious goals and unconscious fantasies about their child. These trends emerging in the parent/analyst Field can readily become a significant source of associative material for the analyst in the child/analyst Field.

By conceptualizing collateral parent work from a Field Theory perspective, the analyst can shift his or her own perspective from a developmentally oriented guidance model to one where the analyst hears the parents' concerns as here-and-now commentary on their emotional state and on the unconscious communication with the analyst, shaping the 'illness' of the Field. This constellation provides opportunities for unsaturated interpretive work and, with it, the metabolization of proto-emotions, expanded narrative co-constructions and emotional transformations. In working with parents, the analyst's association to his or her encounters with the child, to the developmental history or to other pieces of information would be viewed as commentary on the dyadic interchange with the parents per se, influencing the analyst to integrate the joint experience with the parents and offer emotionally salient unsaturated reflections to them. This may serve to better contain the inevitable pressures on the analyst to offer concrete fixes to complex and long-standing problems, a common feature in a reality-oriented perspective and a developmentally oriented guidance approach. Field Theory provides a useful means for conceptualizing the parents' communications to and interactions with the analyst regarding their primary concerns and perspectives on their child. To the extent that a shared unconscious fantasy emerges between parents and analyst, there is an opportunity for greater understanding and transformation in the parents and in their impasses with their child.

Field Theory applied to the child analytic work puts emphasis on the dyadic bi-personal interchange between analyst and child. From this point of view, the analyst's associations to explicit parental wishes, desires and opinions and to unconscious developments in the parent/analyst Field serve to inform the analyst of the unfolding unconscious fantasies mobilized in the dyad with the child. This would suggest a movement toward representation of unthought thoughts and unmetabolized emotions and would provide opportunities for formulation, integration, interpretation and eventual transformation. Field Theory, as applied to child clinical work, provides a means to conceptualize cross-treatment influences and to listen to such influences as valuable commentary within the boundaries of each Field experience.

References

Badoni, M. (2002). Parents and their child – And the analyst in the middle: Working with a transgenerational mandate. *International Journal of Pscyhoanalysis*, 83 (5): 1111–1131.

Baranger, M. and Baranger, W. (1961–1962). The analytic situation as a dynamic Field. *International Journal of Pscyhoanalysis*, 89 (4): 795–826.

Baranger, M. and Baranger, W. (2009). *The Work of Confluence, Listening and Interpreting in the Psychoanalytic Field*. Ed. by L.G. Fiorini. London: Karnac.

Bleger, J. (1967). Pscyho-Analysis of the Psycho-Analytic Frame. *International Journal of Psychoanalysis*, 48: 511–519.

Brady, M. (2019). Book Review: *Field Theory in Child and Adolescent Psychoanalysis: Understanding by and Reacting to Unexpected Developments*. By E. Molinari. *International Journal of Pscyhoanalysis*, 100: 415–418.

Ferro, A. (1999). *The Bi-Personal Field*. New York and London: Routledge.

Ferro, A. (2018). *Dream Model of the Mind in Contemporary Bionian Theory and Technique in Psychoanalysis*. New York and Abingdon: Routledge. pp. 114–148.

Isaacs Elmhirst, S. (1988). The Kleinian setting for child analysis. *International Review of Psychoanalysis*, 15 (1): 5–12.

Molinari, E. (2013a). The anteroom: A camera obscura for grasping aspects invisible in the classical setting. *Psychoanalytic Quarterly*, 82 (4): 811–827.

Molinari, E. (2013b). The use of child drawings to explore the dual group analytic Field in child analysis. *International Journal of Pscyhoanalysis*, 94 (2): 293–312.

Molinari, E. (2017). *Field Theory in Child and Adolescent Psychoanalysis: Understanding and Reacting to Unexpected Developments*. Abingdon and New York: Routledge.

Ogden, T.H. (2005). *The Art of Psychoanalysis: Dreaming Undreamt Dreams and Interrupted Cries*. Abingdon: Routledge.

Ogden, T.H. (2008). *Rediscovering Psychoanalysis: Thinking, and Dreaming, Learning and Forgetting*. Abingdon: Routledge.

Chapter 9

Coda

The Field of the future, the future of the Field

Howard B. Levine

Bion (1970) saw the psychic apparatus as a late evolutionary acquisition, the purpose of which was to help us accommodate to and withstand what he felt were the inherently traumatic experiences of being sentient and alive. He ascribed the means for doing so to alpha function – originally referred to in *Cogitations* (Bion, 1992) as 'dreamwork alpha' – and elaborated his theory of container/contained (Bion, 1962, 1970), noting that as a species, our capacity for containment was rudimentary at best. His formulation of waking dream thoughts, a full-time process that took place both day and night, attested to the relentlessness of the regulatory need with which we face every moment of our lives. This line of thinking extended that of Freud (1920), who had speculated that the 'excitation' of being alive had induced in the first living micro-organism a 'reflexive' response aimed at returning to the insensate 'peacefulness' of the inanimate state. Freud (1920) referred to this response as The Nirvana Principle, implicated it in the clinical phenomena of the Repetition Compulsion, in the play of children in the search for mastery and ultimately suggested that returning to a previous state or level of organization was an implicit and essential characteristic of the drives, Eros as well as Thanatos.

Implicit in the thinking of both authors was a belief that human existence and the uncomfortable emotions it can elicit are a full-time, lifelong problem for us all. While the struggle to stay attuned to the pain and discomfort produced by the limitations of reality may be momentarily put aside, they are ever present and never settled. The clinical urgency of this struggle can be seen in Freud's (1911) descriptions of the conflicts that occur between the Pleasure Principle and the Reality Principle and in Bion's (1965, 1970) assertion that there are two kinds of patients, those who can bear the pain of frustration and form thoughts and think about the frustrating object in its absence, and those who cannot.

If the exigency of regulatory need is a *raison d'etre* of psychic functioning and the means to achieve regulation reflects the action of waking dream thoughts (alpha function), then psychoanalytic attention must be paid to the oneiric dimension of being and the subjective level of created personal

DOI: 10.4324/9781003168034-9

meanings that we call psychic reality. Nino Ferro has attempted to clinically operationalize our understanding and intersubjective access to that dimension in his formulations of Field Theory. The essays in this book reflect and respond to Ferro's recognition that Bion has offered us a somewhat different and certainly more optimistic perspective of the unconscious than many of us encountered in our more classical analytic formations. For Bion, raw, existential Experience[1] as a thing-in-itself, as O, is infinite and unknowable. Capital E Experience is the infinite domain of concrete 'facts' that are in need of transformational process to be made into 'knowable' experience – $(T(O) \rightarrow K)$ – that is, made finite, bounded and meaningful at a personal, subjective level.

The most important of these unknowable 'facts' are our initial, raw emotions, which Bion (1963) qualified as beta elements. These may have sensorial presence and some degree of signification, but are not yet 'thinkable' or developed to the point where we might call them symbols. Beta elements cannot be thought with or thought about. They are, in their initial state, only amenable to suppression or evacuation.[2] But while evacuation serves the immediate aim of discharge and tension reduction, in the context of a suitable intersubjective relationship, in the presence of a more developed, receptive mind, the evacuation may also be seen to contain a covert 'call for help' in regard to both metabolization of the heretofore uncontainable – this is the communicative aspect of projective identification – and in the strengthening of one's future capacities for autonomously creating containment – the development of one's own alpha function.

Bion (1970) shifts a main axis of psychoanalytic emphasis from 'conscious vs. unconscious' to that of 'finite vs. infinite'. At every moment, the domain of raw existential Experience is infinite, but the capacity of the human psyche to encompass and make sense of that experience is not. As an approximation, we might say that the psyche is three dimensional, corresponding to our mind's capacity to comprehend and approximate what in the ordinary, non-quantum physical world we call three-dimensional space – perhaps four dimensional, if we include the dimension of time. The contrast between Experience and that part of it that has the potential to become knowable, trying to capture and hold an infinity of contents in a finite dimensional container, creates a strain of unimaginable force. This can only be posited, never fully 'felt' or 'known' and may only be approximated by expressions, such as: 'an annihilating, centrifugal force that threatens to fragment and destroy one's mind, unless it is reined in and buffered by some kind of organization or barrier'. While this expression is a metaphor for the 'black hole' of nameless dread, it also marks the potentially more optimistic vision of an infinite unconscious that consists of elements which, if they can to some degree be contained and transformed, offers us an ever expanding, inexhaustible domain of great personal potential, one that is continuously available for further development and growth.

Whereas Freud taught us that the night dreams of normal and neurotic patients, those sequences of images (alpha elements) that are evoked during REM sleep, may have symbolic meanings that may be uncovered and constructed by a process of free association and interpretation, Bion taught us that there is a whole, unending universe of beta elements that are in potential need of transformation into waking dream thoughts, the way that the Six Characters in Pirandello's famous play are in search of an Author. From this perspective, Ferro's metaphor of the Field opens up a perspective on the analytic relationship and interaction as an oneiric space of emotions, dreams and 'characters' that are continually appearing and being assembled to await construction and coherence via the processes of assignment of meaning, subjectivization, objectalization (Green, 2005), temporal ordering, narrative construction and all the operations served by the apparatus for thinking thoughts and the apparatus for dreaming dreams that are included in the short-hand formula, container/contained.

As Nino has often implied in his many books, papers and conference talks, the Field is the metaphorical space in which emotions and other beta elements can begin to 'live', to 'dance'. They assemble themselves into innumerable narratives that are the stuff of coherence that will solidify and create our identities and give meaning to our lives. Moment to moment, the words, gestures, feelings and actions of the analytic couple, individually and shared, unconsciously 'cast' the characters and proto-characters of the Field upon the dream stage of the setting and from this, depending upon our analytic theory and vertex, a drama may be seen to unfold from which the multiple perspectives of external reality, internal reality, transference as displaced objects, feelings and relations from the past, etc. may be discerned, or, perhaps more accurately, inferred – or, in Freud's (1937) term, constructed.

From the Field perspective, the oneiric space of the analysis is turned into a transitional zone in which the characters and movements of the Field arise spontaneously and unwittingly from the minds of both participants and constitute a separate, metaphoric 'reality'. The psychic reality of the Field is such that from the Field perspective, one cannot say to whom, analyst or patient, an emotion, character, movement, etc. belongs. Each is a property of the Field. This vertex valorizes an important aspect of the analyst's subjective response to the here-and-now of the process (so-called countertransference) as an actualization (casting) of the Field. (Recall Paula Heimann's (1950) assertion that the analyst's countertransference is an aspect of the *patient's* character.)

If we now recall the plea for regulatory assistance inherent in the patient's unwitting contributions to the force, direction and shape of casting, then we have a perspective in which the analytic interaction and process becomes a giant Winnicottian Squiggle Game, in which the emergent forms are transformations and containers of previously unmetabolized forces from which each member of the analytic pair is seeking transformational relief. Although we may note from a different perspective that the contributions are not fully symmetrical – the greater need for containment and regulation is usually inherent in the patient, and the analyst's theoretical and ethical commitments dictate that he or she is there in the service of the patient's emotional needs – the limitations that extend to all of us by virtue of our humanity imply that to some degree, the analyst will also be the potential recipient of transformational relief in the course of the analytic process.

In regard to analytic technique, Nino has drawn our attention to the importance of containment and the transformational power of the analyst's interventions. The designation of *unsaturated* interpretations adds an evocative and playful dimension to the certainty of communication of fixed (saturated) meaning. It also emphasizes the importance of analytic process – the verbal Squiggle Game – instead of an exclusive and relentless search for hidden contents. This orientation reflects Nino's background as a child analyst versed and immersed in the dimension of play therapy and his interest in the realms of linguistic theory and narratology.

In an online conference on The Post-Bionian Field Theory of Antonino Ferro, organized by the Antonio Santamaria Foundation in Mexico City, 2020, Nino introduced his newest ideas to the audience and charged us with the task of exploring and developing them, adding ideas of our own and, in so doing, helping to move psychoanalysis and Field Theory even further forward into the twenty-first century (Ferro, 2020). He began by reminding us that just as Freud had taught us to recognize that there were other worlds – most notably the world of the dynamic, repressed unconscious – beyond the manifest world of consciousness, so Bion taught us that there were infinite universes – the unrepresented, not yet formed, emergent, unstructured unconscious – beyond our own.

Referencing Bion's Grid – a complex, often controversial and hard to understand instrument that Bion devised for the tracking of transformations and movement within the session – and Bion's suggestion that one could develop many different Grids to track movements and psychic development within a session at many levels and from many different points of view, Nino reminded us of quantum physics, and suggested that we could begin to think of psychic multi-verses that existed alongside the now well-travelled and still useful psychoanalytic dimensions that we have familiarized ourselves with in the past 130 years. Could we, perhaps, usefully map out a domain of negative reveries and reversed alpha function and construct a 'minus Grid'? Or create a Grid of negative capability? The possibilities, he suggested, might be as infinite as Experience itself.

He spoke of the Italian painter, Lucio Fontana, who painted images and then literally gouged cuts into the canvas, so that we might look into and behind the image and the canvas that we were observing. This was an opening to another world, unseen, unknown and yet always present. If we could do the same in an analysis, what else might we discover? If the Grid cannot contain the forces present, if the container ruptures what might we find? A 'dark Grid' analogous to the 'dark web' of the internet? A secret space? Perhaps the secret space of Winnicott's True Self that always remains hidden? The infinite? As in the movie *Waterworld*, would we need to develop metaphorical gills in order to 'breathe' and survive in the exploration of this dark world?

Clearly, he left us with a great deal to think about and a great deal to do. But with an expectation of excitement and adventure. Among his last words were these: 'When we lose the capacity to dream, we fall into the negative Grid. We stop dreaming and begin the negative Grid'. If we fall out of our now comfortable universe, into the multi-verses of the unknown, what will we discover? What words can we find to describe our discoveries to others and to ourselves? Will this help define the psychoanalysis of the twenty-first century?

In response to a series of questions from the audience, Nino added:

> Concepts such as the negative Grid, the negative Field, parallel universes and multi-verses are yet to be fully explored and endowed with meaning, and may therefore be regarded as tools more than concepts – tools which may allow us to explore unknown meanings and worlds and spaces … It is by using these new tools that we will come to understand them more. We might liken them to a spaceship that will take us somewhere. We still don't know where that might be or what we might find once we get there.
>
> (Ferro, 2020)

What Nino is asking us to do is to postpone a final closure of meaning, insisting instead upon unsaturated, open interpretations – and an open-ended psychoanalytic theory – that call upon the patient to engage in imaginative work that evokes further dialogue that can then develop along unexpected lines. This creates a welcoming atmosphere in the analysis and lends itself to the perception of nuance and the discovery of the pleasure that is inherent in the 'psychoanalytic game'. As he himself put it once in a discussion:

> There is a value to allowing recourse to allusive (from the Latin *ad* + *ludere*, which means 'play'), evocative and elliptical rhetoric, that suggests a direction, without resolving meaning completely, leaving space to the other, space for the unsaid, even to reticence, to an eloquent silence that is neither opaque nor closed in on itself, a silence that creates a concave, receptive space, the opposite of noise and not of speech, open to the un-fore-seen and to the un-known of the unconscious.

The patient may then experience the analyst as someone who puts up with uncertainty, contradictions, complexity; who is able to tolerate not being able to understand everything at once, who is also able to look out over the abyss of insignificance of the human condition, but who nonetheless has a method which he trusts will help him acquire and help others acquire a new narrative competence and growth of thought with respect to all of this.

Described in this way, this analytic attitude may seem minimalist, but it is far from being oracular or opposed to knowing; nor is it dogmatizing or aestheticizing. The analyst takes maximum responsibility with respect to the patient, knowing that, as Bion never tires of repeating, pain, fear and danger are necessarily present in the theatre of analysis. In this way, the truth of the fundamental solitude of the human condition should emerge, and ideally, at the conclusion of the analysis when patients take their leave, they should take with them the secret of the illusory nature of reality, a sense of the transient nature of things or, as Searles (1961) would put it, the acceptance of the idea of the inevitability of suffering and death. This is, after all, the lucid pessimism that Freud showed, or rather 'the gentleness of a well-tempered skepticism that is devoid of any idealization of the negative' (Ferro, personal communication, 2018).

Notes

1 I shall refer to the unprocessed, untransformed, raw existential 'experience' of being alive in the world as Experience – with a capital E – and to the 'experience' of everyday speech that can be known, thought of and talked about as experience with a small e.
2 To avoid confusion, Bion categorized emotions as beta elements, implying that unless and until transformed into alpha elements, these raw emotions might be felt as concrete sensations – sensorial disturbances – but were not yet qualifiable as specific affects that could be linked to ideational elements to make what in common parlance are called 'thoughts'. For Bion, ideation not drawn from emotional experience – i.e. without linked affect – is intellectualization; true thought has its roots in instinctual manifestations, growing into imaginative elaboration. (See Green, 2000, p. 80.)

References

Bion, W.R. (1962). *Learning From Experience.* London: Heinemann.
Bion, W.R. (1963). *Elements of Psycho-Analysis.* London: Karnac.
Bion, W.R. (1965). *Transformations.* London: Karnac.
Bion, W.R. (1970). *Attention and Interpretation.* New York: Basic Books.
Bion, W.R. (1992). *Cogitations.* London: Karnac.
Ferro, A. (2020). Field Theory. Presented at The Post-Bionian Field Theory of Antonino Ferro, an online conference hosted by the Antonio Santamaria Foundation, Mexico City, November 15.
Freud, S. (1911). *Formulations on the two principles of mental functioning.* S.E. 12. pp. 215–226.
Freud, S. (1920). *Beyond the pleasure principle.* S.E. 18. pp. 1–64.
Freud, S. (1937). *Constructions in analysis.* S.E. 23. pp. 257–269.
Green, A. (2000). *Andre Green at the Squiggle Foundation.* London: Karnac.
Green, A. (2005). *Key Ideas for a Contemporary Psychoanalysis.* New York and Abingdon: Routledge.
Heimann, P. (1950). On counter-transference. *International Journal of Psychoanalysis,* 31: 81–84.
Searles, H. (1961). Anxiety concerning change, as seen in the psychotherapy of schizophrenic patients – With particular reference to the sense of personal identity. *International Journal of Psychoanalysis,* 42: 74–85.

Index

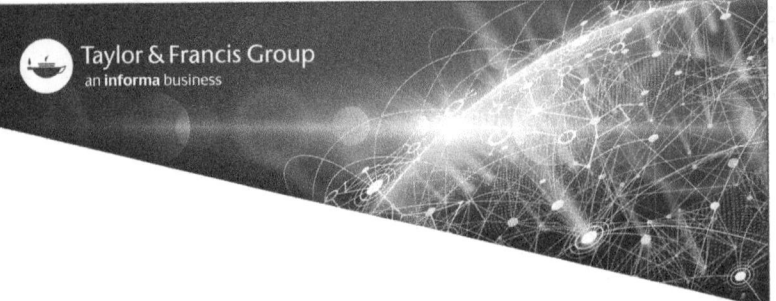
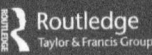
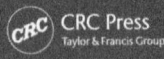